Study Guide

Understanding Pharmacology

Essentials for Medication Safety, Second Edition

M. Linda Workman, PhD, RN, FAAN
Linda LaCharity, PhD, RN

Study Guide prepared by:

Jennifer Ponto, RN, BSN
Instructor
Department of Vocational Nursing
South Plains College
Levelland, Texas

ELSEVIER

ELSEVIER

3251 Riverport Lane
Maryland Heights, MO 63043

STUDY GUIDE FOR UNDERSTANDING PHARMACOLOGY:
ESSENTIALS FOR MEDICATION SAFETY, SECOND EDITION

ISBN: 978-0-3233-9494-9

Content Strategist: Nancy O'Brien
Content Development Manager: Ellen Wurm-Cutter
Associate Content Development Specialist: Katie Gutierrez
Publishing Services Manager: Deepthi Unni
Senior Project Manager: Radhika Sivalingam

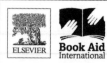

Working together
to grow libraries in
developing countries

www.elsevier.com • www.bookaid.org

Printed in the United States of America
Last digit is the print number: 9 8 7 6 5 4 3 2 1

To the Student

This study guide was created to assist you in achieving the objectives of each chapter in the second edition of *Understanding Pharmacology: Essentials for Medication Safety*, and establishing a solid base of knowledge in pharmacology. Completing the exercises in each chapter in this guide will help to reinforce the material studied in the textbook and learned in class. Such reinforcement also helps students to be successful on licensure exams.

STUDY HINTS FOR ALL STUDENTS

Ask Questions!
There are no stupid questions. If you do not know something or are not sure, you need to find out. Other people may be wondering the same thing but may be too shy to ask. The answer could mean life or death to your patient. That is certainly more important than feeling embarrassed about asking a question.

Chapter Objectives
At the beginning of each chapter in the textbook are objectives that you should have mastered when you finish studying that chapter. Write these objectives in your notebook, leaving a blank space after each. Fill in the answers as you find them while reading the chapter. Review to make sure your answers are correct and complete. Use these answers when you study for tests. This should also be done for separate course objectives that your instructor has listed in your class syllabus.

Key Terms
At the beginning of each chapter in the textbook are key terms that you will encounter as you read the chapter. The key terms are in color the first time they appear significantly in the chapter. Phonetic pronunciations are provided for terms that students might find difficult to pronounce. The terms that were assigned simple phonetic pronunciations were selected because they are either (1) difficult medical, nursing, or scientific terms or (2) other words that may be difficult for students to pronounce. The goal is to help the student reader with limited proficiency in English to develop a greater command of the pronunciation of scientific and nonscientific English terminology. It is hoped that a more general competency in the understanding and use of medical and scientific language may result.

Key Points
Use the Key Points at the end of each chapter in the textbook to help with review for exams.

Reading Hints
When reading each chapter in the textbook, look at the subject headings to learn what each section is about. Read first for the general meaning. Then reread parts you did not understand. It may help to read those parts aloud. Carefully read the information given in each table and study each figure and its caption.

Concepts
While studying, put difficult concepts into your own words to see if you understand them. Check this understanding with another student or the instructor. Write these in your notebook.

Class Notes
When taking lecture notes in class, leave a large margin on the left side of each notebook page and write only on right-hand pages, leaving all left-hand pages blank. Look over your lecture notes soon after each class, while your memory is fresh. Fill in missing words, complete sentences and ideas, and underline key phrases, definitions, and concepts. At the top of each page, write the topic of that page. In the left margin,

write the key word for that part of your notes. On the opposite left-hand page, write a summary or outline that combines material from both the textbook and the lecture. These can be your study notes for review.

Study Groups

Form a study group with some other students so you can help one another. Practice speaking and reading aloud. Ask questions about material you are not sure about. Work together to find answers.

References for Improving Study Skills

Good study skills are essential for achieving your goals in nursing. Time management, efficient use of study time, and a consistent approach to studying are all beneficial. There are various study methods for reading a textbook and for taking class notes. Some methods that have proven helpful can be found in *Saunders Student Nurse Planner: A Guide to Success in Nursing School.* This book contains helpful information on test taking and preparing for clinical experiences. It includes an example of a "time map" for planning study time and a blank form that the student can use to formulate a personal time map.

ADDITIONAL STUDY HINTS FOR ENGLISH AS SECOND-LANGUAGE (ESL) STUDENTS

Vocabulary

If you find a nontechnical word you do not know (e.g., *drowsy*), try to guess its meaning from the sentence (e.g., *With electrolyte imbalance, the patient may feel fatigued and drowsy*). If you are not sure of the meaning, or if it seems particularly important, look it up in the dictionary.

Vocabulary Notebook

Keep a small alphabetized notebook or address book in your pocket or purse. Write down new nontechnical words you read or hear along with their meanings and pronunciations. Write each word under its initial letter so you can find it easily, as in a dictionary. For words you do not know or for words that have a different meaning in nursing, write down how they are used and sound. Look up their meanings in a dictionary or ask your instructor or first-language buddy. Then write the different meanings or usages that you have found in your book, including the nursing meaning. Continue to add new words as you discover them. For example:

primary
- of most importance; main: *the primary problem or disease*
- the first one; elementary: *primary school*

secondary
- of less importance; resulting from another problem or disease: *a secondary symptom*
- the second one: *secondary school (in the United States, high school)*

First Language Buddy

ESL students should find a first-language buddy – another student who is a native speaker of English and who is willing to answer questions about word meanings, pronunciations, and culture. Maybe your buddy would also like to learn about your language and culture. This could help in his or her learning experience as well.

Contents

Drug Regulation, Actions, and Responses

LEARNING ACTIVITIES

Terminology Review

Match each definition with its corresponding term. (Use each term only once; not all terms will be used.)

_____ 1. Hormones, enzymes, growth factors, and other chemicals made by the body that change the activity of cells

_____ 2. Drugs that are man-made (synthetic) or derived from another species; not made by the human body

_____ 3. The science and study of drugs and their actions on living animals

_____ 4. Drug action that is intended to kill a cell or an organism

_____ 5. A substance that blocks the receptor site of a cell, preventing the naturally occurring substance from binding to the receptor

_____ 6. A substance that activates the receptor site of a cell and mimics the actions of naturally occurring drugs

_____ 7. The length of time a drug is present in the blood at or above the level needed to produce an effect or response

_____ 8. Movement of a drug from the outside of the body to the inside through the skin or mucous membranes

_____ 9. Movement of a drug from the outside of the body to the inside of the body by injection

_____ 10. Movement of drugs from the outside of the body to the inside using the gastrointestinal tract

_____ 11. The extent that a drug absorbed into the bloodstream spreads into the three body water compartments

_____ 12. The removal of drugs from the body accomplished by certain body systems

_____ 13. Movement of a drug from the outside of the body into the bloodstream

_____ 14. The smallest amount of drug necessary in the blood or target tissue to result in a measurable intended action

_____ 15. The lowest or minimal blood drug level

A. Agonist
B. Antagonist
C. Metabolism
D. Elimination
E. Absorption
F. Distribution
G. Extrinsic drugs
H. Intrinsic drugs
I. Peak
J. Trough
K. Minimum effective concentration
L. Duration of action
M. Cytotoxic
N. Enteral route
O. Parenteral route
P. Percutaneous route
Q. Pharmacodynamics
R. Pharmacology

Matching

Match the effect or response with its correct description. (Answers may only be used once.)

_____ 16. After taking an antibiotic, a patient developed an itchy rash.

_____ 17. After taking a sleeping pill, a patient was asleep for 6 hours.

_____ 18. A patient developed pseudomembranous colitis after taking antibiotics for 2 weeks.

_____ 19. A patient felt drowsy after taking an antihistamine.

_____ 20. A 72-year-old patient stayed awake all night after taking a sleeping pill. He reported feeling nervous.

_____ 21. A patient developed hemolytic anemia while taking a drug for malaria.

A. Paradoxical effect
B. Allergic response
C. Side effect
D. Adverse drug effect
E. Idiosyncratic (personal) response
F. Therapeutic effect

Matching: Life Span Categories

Match the life span category to the correct issue or description. (Answers may be used more than once.)

_____ 22. Greater proportion of total body water

_____ 23. Need to avoid drugs that are teratogens

_____ 24. Reduced blood flow to the liver and other body areas

_____ 25. Reduced numbers of red blood cells and tissue oxygenation

_____ 26. May need a higher drug dose in terms of milligrams per kilogram of body weight

_____ 27. Placenta is not a perfect barrier

_____ 28. More likely to have a paradoxical reaction to a drug

_____ 29. Reduced rate of drug elimination

_____ 30. Problematic for drugs needed to manage chronic disorders

A. Pediatric consideration
B. Pregnancy/breastfeeding consideration
C. Older adult consideration

Identification: Intrinsic and Extrinsic Drugs

Specify whether each item below is an intrinsic substance (I) or an extrinsic substance (E).

_____ 31. Insulin secreted by the pancreas

_____ 32. An antihypertensive drug

_____ 33. Endorphins secreted by the body

_____ 34. Morphine sulfate given for pain

Identification: Drug Administration Routes

Specify below which drug administration route is described. Then specify whether the route is percutaneous, parenteral, or enteral.

_____ _____ 35. A tablet that is swallowed through the mouth

_____ _____ 36. A patch that is applied to the skin

_____ _____ 37. Injection into the fatty tissue below the skin

_____ _____ 38. Injection into the bloodstream through a vein

_____ _____ 39. Inhaled as a spray through the nose

_____ _____ 40. Injection into a muscle

_____ _____ 41. A liquid that is swallowed through the mouth

_____ _____ 42. An injection into a joint

_____ _____ 43. A cream placed in the lowest 1.5 inches of the rectum

_____ _____ 44. Medication placed under the tongue

Fill in the Blank

45. The _____, _____, _____, _____, _____, and _____ have the authority to write a drug prescription.

46. Disease of the _____ may affect drug metabolism.

47. A patient with severe kidney disease may have difficulty with drug _____.

48. After the last dose of a drug is given, a drug is considered eliminated after _____ half-lives have passed.

49. Newborn infants may have a slower rate of metabolism than an adult because the liver's _____ system is not yet fully active.

50. Infants have a(n) _____ proportion of total body water than adults.

MEDICATION SAFETY PRACTICE

Identify the correct drug pregnancy category (A, B, C, D, or X) for each description. (Each category will be used only once.)

_____ 1. Drugs in this category have been shown to have an increased risk for birth defects or other problems in the fetus, but the drugs may be given if the benefits of treatment outweigh the risk.

_____ 2. Drugs in this category are not to be given to women who are pregnant.

_____ 3. Drugs in this category do not have an increased risk for birth defects or problems in the fetus.

_____ 4. There have been no adequate studies in pregnant women, but animal studies have shown an increased risk for birth defects or other problems in the fetus.

_____ 5. There have been no adequate studies in pregnant women, but animal studies have not shown an increased risk for birth defects or other problems in the fetus.

_____ 6. When reviewing an order for a high-alert drug, what is the best action to be taken before administering it?

PRACTICE QUIZ

_____ 1. A patient has been taking an opioid for severe pain for 3 days. This morning he says he is constipated. How is this effect described?
   A. Intended effect
   B. Side effect
   C. Adverse effect
   D. Paradoxical effect

2. Who is responsible for teaching patients about their drug therapy? *(Select all that apply.)*
   _____ A. Nurse
   _____ B. Unit secretary
   _____ C. Prescriber
   _____ D. Pharmacist
   _____ E. Nursing assistant

_____ 3. Which describes the name of a drug that is created by the United States Adopted Name council, is relatively short and simple, and is not capitalized when written?
   A. Trade name
   B. Proprietary name
   C. Generic name
   D. Brand name

_____ 4. The student is reviewing principles of pharmacology in preparation for a class, and is reading about the differences between intrinsic and extrinsic drugs. What is an example of an intrinsic drug?
   A. An oral drug taken to lower blood glucose levels
   B. Adrenalin secreted by the adrenal gland
   C. Intravenous opioids given to reduce pain
   D. Inhaled bronchodilators for asthma relief

_____ 5. A drug is administered that will cause the same response as an intrinsic drug when it binds to the receptor of a cell. Which term best describes the action of the drug administered?
   A. Agonist
   B. Antagonist
   C. Cytotoxic
   D. Paradoxical

6. A patient is being monitored for an allergic or anaphylactic reaction after the first dose of an antibiotic. Which assessment finding(s) may indicate an allergic or anaphylactic reaction? *(Select all that apply.)*
____ A. Skin rash
____ B. Difficulty breathing
____ C. Hives on the skin
____ D. High blood pressure
____ E. Swelling of the mouth or throat
____ F. Bounding pulse

____ 7. A dose of medication is to be administered sublingually. Which comment best explains the purpose of this route to a patient or family member?
A. "The medication enters the bloodstream via the gastrointestinal tract."
B. "The medication enters the bloodstream via the tissues under the skin."
C. "The medication moves through muscles into the bloodstream."
D. "The medication moves through oral membranes into the bloodstream."

____ 8. A patient is receiving an intravenous injection of a pain medication. What is an advantage of the intravenous route?
A. The drug goes straight to the liver for the first-pass effect.
B. The drug enters the bloodstream more quickly than the other routes.
C. The intravenous route is safer than the oral route.
D. Intravenous drugs are less expensive than oral drugs.

____ 9. A patient who has one kidney is receiving morning medications. When assessing the patient for drug effects, the patient having only one kidney may result in which problem?
A. Drugs may take longer to be eliminated.
B. Drugs may take a shorter time to be eliminated.
C. Drug metabolism may be increased.
D. Drug metabolism may be decreased.

____ 10. A patient has received a 500-mg dose of medication that has a half-life of 8 hours. How much drug is in the patient's bloodstream 16 hours from the time the medication was administered?
A. 250 mg
B. 125 mg
C. 62.5 mg
D. 31.25 mg

____ 11. When administering drugs to infants and children, it is important to remember which principle of drug therapy?
A. Most medication doses for infants are often higher in proportion than adult doses.
B. Toddlers, preschool and school-age children, and adolescents usually have lower rates of metabolism than adults.
C. An infant's kidneys will concentrate more water than an adult's kidneys.
D. Water-soluble drugs are eliminated more rapidly in infants and young children than they are in adults.

____ 12. An older adult is experiencing heart failure. Heart failure may cause what effect on the drugs that this patient is taking?
A. The distribution of the drugs will be decreased.
B. The metabolism of the drugs will be increased.
C. The drugs will be absorbed more slowly.
D. Heart failure will not have an effect on the drugs.

____ 13. A health care instructor is teaching a class about drug therapy and pregnancy. During which stage of pregnancy is the risk of drug therapy causing birth defects highest?
A. Weeks 1 and 2 of pregnancy
B. Weeks 3 through 8 of pregnancy
C. Weeks 9 through 20 of pregnancy
D. The last 2 weeks of pregnancy

____ 14. A patient asks about taking an herbal supplement to prevent colds. What is the best response?
   A. "Herbal supplements are safe, so you should be fine."
   B. "Just make sure you take this herbal product at least 2 hours after your morning medications."
   C. "Let's discuss this with your prescriber or pharmacist, as there could be interactions."
   D. "You should never take herbal products with your other medications."

15. The nurse's role in drug therapy includes which action(s)? (*Select all that apply.*)
   ____ A. Select and order specific drugs.
   ____ B. Dispense prescribed drugs.
   ____ C. Administer prescribed drugs to the patient.
   ____ D. Teach patients about ordered drugs.
   ____ E. Know the purpose and adverse effects of drugs.

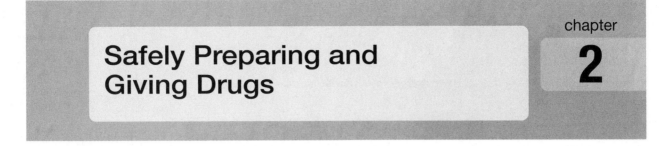

Safely Preparing and Giving Drugs

LEARNING ACTIVITIES

Crossword Puzzle: The Eight Rights of Safe Drug Administration

Each clue reflects a problem with one of the six rights of safe drug administration. Complete the puzzle by identifying the "rights" that are described.

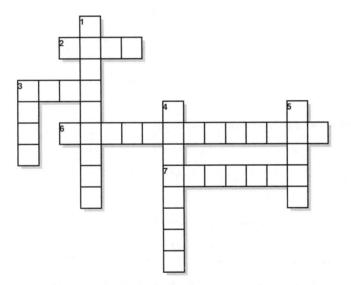

Across

2. The nurse was interrupted during morning medication rounds by an emergency. As a result, doses of morning medications were delayed by 3 hours.
3. The nurse reads the order for "Celebrex," then looks in the drug dispensing cabinet and pulls out "Celexa."
6. At the beginning of a new shift, the nurse sees that a medication that was due 2 hours ago was not signed off on the medication administration record. However, the patient insists that he did receive the medication.
7. During medication rounds, the nurse discovers that the patient is not wearing an identification wristband.

Down

1. A patient is receiving an antibiotic, but actually has a viral infection only.
3. The prescriber gives a verbal order for "IV Lasix, now."
4. A patient says, "I don't know why I even bother taking this antidepressant. I'm still feeling depressed."
5. The nurse is reviewing orders written by the prescriber. One order states, "Give Tylenol, 650 mg, every 4 hours as needed for pain."

Matching

Match the drug order with the correct drug order type. (Each type will be used only once.)

_____ 1. Levothyroxine, 50 mcg, PO daily

_____ 2. Valium, 5 mg, IV 30 minutes before the procedure

_____ 3. Morphine, 2 mg, IV push every 3 hours as needed for pain

_____ 4. Lasix, 40 mg, PO immediately

A. STAT
B. Standing
C. Single dose
D. PRN

Before or After?

For each action listed, state whether the action is Before or After giving a drug. (Note: Some actions may be done before AND after.)

_____ 5. Ask the patient about drug allergies.

_____ 6. Check the residual amount of tube feeding remaining in the patient's stomach.

_____ 7. Check the placement of the feeding tube.

_____ 8. Flush the feeding tube with at least 50 mL of water.

_____ 9. Ask the patient to gently blow his or her nose.

_____ 10. Monitor the patient for therapeutic and adverse effects.

_____ 11. Ask the patient to empty his or her bladder.

_____ 12. Remove the old patch and any trace of previous doses.

_____ 13. Check the patient's identification wristband.

_____ 14. For rectally administered drugs, remind the patient to remain on his or her side for 20 minutes.

_____ 15. Pull the ear lobe up and out for children older than age 3 and adults.

_____ 16. Wash your hands.

_____ 17. Measure the liquid drug in a calibrated device.

_____ 18. Document the drugs that were given.

_____ 19. Select an appropriate needle for the injection.

Fill in the Blank

Complete each statement that describes how each type of injection is given.

20. Intradermal drugs are injected _____. The length and gauge of the needle is _____ and the amount injected is _____ to _____ mL. The needle is inserted at a _____-degree angle, and the bevel is facing _____.

21. Subcutaneous drugs are injected _____. The length and gauge of the needle is _____. The needle is inserted at a _____-degree angle for most patients, but a _____-degree angle may be needed for obese patients. Typical amounts for these injections are _____ to _____ mL.

22. Intramuscular drugs are injected _____. Needles for these injections are _____ inches in length, and _____ gauge in size. The needle is inserted at a _____-degree angle for the injection. For an adult, the maximum amount that can be injected is _____ mL; for infants and children the amount is _____ mL.

True or False: Drug Administration

State whether each statement is True or False. If the statement is false, rewrite it to make it true.

_____ 23. Aspirate by pulling back on the plunger of the syringe after injecting a subcutaneous dose of heparin or insulin.

_____ 24. Intradermal drugs are given in the inner part of the forearm.

_____ 25. Remove the needle and discard the needle and syringe, without injecting the drug, if blood is seen in the syringe when aspirating during an intramuscular injection.

_____ 26. Place the sublingual tablet between the cheek and the molar teeth of the upper jaw.

_____ 27. When giving eardrops to a child younger than 3 years, pull the ear lobe down and back.

_____ 28. Teach the patient not to swallow or chew a sublingual or buccal tablet while it is dissolving in the mouth.

_____ 29. A drug given by the intravenous route is injected directly into a vein.

_____ 30. The Z-track method for intramuscular (IM) injections is used for all IM injections.

_____ 31. After giving medications, reattach the nasogastric tube to suction.

Matching

Match each intervention to its appropriate drug route. (Drug routes may be used more than once, and not all options may be used.)

_____ 32. Inject into the fatty tissues between the skin and the muscle layers.

_____ 33. Use a 1- to 1.5-inch, 20- to 22-gauge needle for the injection.

_____ 34. Be sure the patient can swallow.

_____ 35. Use a 3/8-inch, 25-gauge needle, and 0.01 to 0.1 mL of fluid for the injection.

_____ 36. Remove the old patch and clean the skin thoroughly.

_____ 37. Have the patient lie down for 15 to 20 minutes after receiving the drug.

_____ 38. Use the Z-track technique when injecting drugs that are irritating.

_____ 39. Check the gastric residual before giving the medication.

_____ 40. Place the tablet between the cheek and the molar teeth of the upper jaw.

_____ 41. Stop the medication if fluid collects in the tissues.

_____ 42. Do not give if the patient is experiencing diarrhea.

_____ 43. Give the injection into the space between the epidermis and the dermis layers of the skin.

_____ 44. Potential injection sites include the deltoid, vastus lateralis, and dorsogluteal areas.

_____ 45. Use a 3/8-inch, 25- to 27-gauge needle with 0.5 to 1 mL of fluid for the injection.

_____ 46. Wash hands.

A. Oral
B. Rectal
C. Intradermal
D. Subcutaneous
E. Intramuscular
F. Nasogastric tube
G. Intravenous
H. Buccal
I. Sublingual
J. Nasal
K. Vaginal
L. Topical/transdermal
M. All routes

MEDICATION SAFETY PRACTICE

For each statement or scenario, identify whether the action is Correct or Incorrect. If incorrect, rewrite the statement to make the action correct.

_____ 1. After giving an injection, the cap is placed back on the needle before placing it into a sharps container.

_____ 2. The patient is in the bathroom when medications are given. The patient asks the health care worker to leave the medications on the bedside table, and the worker does as requested.

_____ 3. The nurse draws up an injection into a syringe, and then asks another health care worker to administer it because a different patient needs to be checked immediately.

_____ 4. The dorsogluteal injection site is selected for an intramuscular injection for an infant.

_____ 5. A drug error was made and immediately reported.

_____ 6. The patient states, "I can't swallow that capsule." The capsule is opened and given to the patient.

_____ 7. The person giving medications stays at the bedside until the drugs are swallowed.

_____ 8. The patient is assisted to the left Sims' position before giving a rectal suppository.

_____ 9. The deltoid site is selected to give a vaccination to a 16-year-old patient.

_____ 10. Before giving an intravenous infusion, the nurse removes all of the air from the tubing.

_____ 11. During medication administration, the patient states, "I don't recognize that pill. Are you sure it is right?" The order is checked before giving the medication.

Are Gloves Needed?

For each drug administration route listed below, mark "Y" for yes if gloves are needed for administration or "N" for no if gloves are not needed.

_____ 12. Oral tablet

_____ 13. Oral liquid

_____ 14. Rectal suppository

_____ 15. Intradermal injection

_____ 16. Subcutaneous injection

_____ 17. Intravenous piggyback drug

_____ 18. Sublingual tablet

_____ 19. Eardrops

_____ 20. Transdermal patch

_____ 21. Vaginal cream

PRACTICE QUIZ

1. A patient, who is new to the unit, is receiving medications. What should be done to ensure that the right patient is receiving the right drugs? *(Select all that apply.)*
   ____ A. Check the patient's name on the wristband.
   ____ B. Ask the patient to state his or her name and birthdate.
   ____ C. Check the patient's birthdate on the wristband.
   ____ D. Check the patient's identification number.
   ____ E. Check the patient's room number.

____ 2. A patient needs an oral dose of acetaminophen every 4 hours if the patient's oral temperature reaches 101.5° F (38.6° C) or greater. This is recognized as which type of order?
   A. PRN
   B. STAT
   C. Single
   D. Standing

____ 3. Prior to drug administration, a dosage calculation is performed. Which is the best action to prevent drug errors?
   A. Use a calculator for the dosage calculation.
   B. Perform the calculation twice.
   C. Check the dosage calculation with a coworker.
   D. Look up the dosage in a drug resource book.

____ 4. The nurse is administering morning medications and assess the patient first. The patient states, "Ever since I started that yellow pill, I've felt dizzy and nauseated." What should the nurse do next?
   A. Assure the patient that this is normal.
   B. Administer the drug.
   C. Wait an hour before giving the drug.
   D. Hold the drug and notify the prescriber.

____ 5. Medications will be administered through a nasogastric tube. When testing with an end-tidal CO_2 detector, the presence of CO_2 is noted. What should be the next action?
   A. Administer the medications.
   B. Flush the tubing with 50 mL of water.
   C. Attach the tubing to suction.
   D. Hold the medications.

____ 6. An intramuscular injection will be given to an adult patient. Upon checking the dosage, the volume of the injection is 3.2 mL. Which action is appropriate?
   A. Give the entire amount in one injection.
   B. Divide the dose and give two injections.
   C. Use the Z-track method to administer the injection.
   D. Hold the injection and notify the prescriber.

____ 7. A patient's family member is preparing to administer a topical cream to a patient's skin. Which action by the family member reflects a need for further teaching?
   A. Performing handwashing and applying gloves before giving the medication
   B. Cleaning the patient's skin before applying the medication
   C. Shaving the patient's hair off the site before applying the medication
   D. Applying a smooth, thin layer to the patient's skin

____ 8. A patient's wife is being taught how to administer eardrops to her husband. Which action by the wife indicates a need for further teaching?
   A. Pulling the ear lobe down and back to give the eardrops
   B. Pulling the ear lobe up and out to give the eardrops
   C. Asking her husband to lie on his side for at least 5 minutes after giving the drops
   D. Administering the drug without letting the ear dropper touch the ear

____ 9. Morning medications have been given to a patient with hypertension. Which immediate action is most appropriate at this time?
   A. Checking the patient's blood pressure
   B. Assessing the patient's pain level
   C. Teaching the patient the purpose of the medication
   D. Documenting the medication given

____ 10. Crushed oral medication will be given to a 3-year-old child. Which statement is appropriate?
   A. "Here is some candy for you!"
   B. "This medicine tastes really good!"
   C. "Would you like to take it with apple juice or fruit punch?"
   D. "Would you like me to mix this in a glass of orange juice?"

Mathematics Review and Introduction to Dosage Calculations

chapter

3

LEARNING ACTIVITIES

Matching: Terminology Review

Match each definition with its corresponding term. (Use each term only once; not all terms will be used.)

_____ 1. The bottom number in a fraction

_____ 2. The top number in a fraction that is divided by the bottom number

_____ 3. The answer to a division problem

_____ 4. The expression of how a number is related to 100

_____ 5. The part of a whole number based on a system of units of 10

_____ 6. An equal mathematic relationship between two sets of numbers

_____ 7. A fraction that has a numerator that is lower than the denominator

_____ 8. A fraction that has a whole number with a fraction attached

_____ 9. A fraction that has been changed to the lowest common denominator

_____ 10. The number to be divided in a division problem

A. Proper fraction
B. Reduced fraction
C. Mixed-number fraction
D. Improper fraction
E. Dividend
F. Divisor
G. Decimal
H. Numerator
I. Denominator
J. Percent
K. Quotient
L. Proportion

Fill in the Blank: Mathematics Review

11. For the fractions listed below, identify the numerator and denominator, and specify whether the fraction is a proper or improper fraction.

   a. $\frac{5}{9}$

   b. $\frac{9}{4}$

   c. $\frac{11}{6}$

   d. $\frac{2}{3}$

12. For the decimal numbers listed below, identify the divisor, the dividend, and the quotient.

   a. $^{36.5}\!\!/_2$

   b. $^{11.4}\!\!/_{5.9}$

   c. $^{30.3}\!\!/_5$

   d. $^{52.5}\!\!/_{4.6}$

13. Change each number below to a fraction.

   a. 9

   b. 552

14. Change each mixed number fraction below to an improper fraction.

   a. $1\,\tfrac{3}{4}$

   b. $5\,\tfrac{1}{3}$

15. Reduce each fraction to its lowest terms.

   a. $^{75}\!\!/_{100}$

   b. $^{99}\!\!/_{126}$

   c. $^{53}\!\!/_{72}$

   d. $^{12}\!\!/_{288}$

16. Calculate the answer to each problem below. If the answer is an improper fraction, convert it to a mixed number fraction.

   a. $\tfrac{2}{3} + \tfrac{5}{3}$

   b. $\tfrac{1}{6} + \tfrac{2}{6} + \tfrac{3}{6} + \tfrac{5}{6}$

   c. $\tfrac{2}{6} + \tfrac{3}{5} + \tfrac{1}{3}$

   d. $\tfrac{6}{8} - \tfrac{4}{8}$

   e. $4\,\tfrac{3}{8} - ^{12}\!\!/_8$

   f. $7\,\tfrac{5}{8} - 2\,\tfrac{1}{5}$

   g. $\tfrac{4}{8} \times \tfrac{1}{3}$

    h. $\frac{1}{8} \times 5\frac{1}{2}$

    i. $7\frac{1}{2} \times 4\frac{1}{5}$

    j. $4 \div \frac{1}{2}$

    k. $\frac{7}{8} \div \frac{1}{3}$

    l. $7\frac{1}{4} \div \frac{3}{5}$

17. Calculate the product or quotient of each problem below.

    a. 0.125×100

    b. 11.4×5.9

    c. $\frac{1}{5} \times 3.8$

    d. $550 \div 0.2$

    e. $1.7 \div 1.7$

    f. $6.5 \div 0.35$

18. Change each fraction below to a decimal.

    a. $\frac{75}{100}$

    b. $\frac{1}{3}$

    c. $\frac{4}{5}$

19. Change each decimal below to a fraction.

    a.   0.25

    b.   0.88

    c.   0.46

20. Calculate the given percentages of each number below.

    a.   1% of 100

    b.   55% of 50

    c.   0.5% of 10

21. Express each problem below as a fractional proportion.

    a. If one batch of cookies yields 12 cookies, then 3 batches of cookies yields 36 cookies.

    b. If 1 mL of filgrastim contains 300 mcg, then 2 mL contains 600 mcg.

MEDICATION SAFETY PRACTICE

1. Which decimal numbers are written correctly? What is wrong with the decimal numbers that are written incorrectly?

    a. .125

    b. .1250

    c. 0.125

    d. 0.1250

    e. 1250.0

2. If a dosage calculation results in the dosage being 1.5 scored tablets, how many tablets will you give? Will you round up or down? Explain your answer.

3. A patient is to receive 40 mg of promethazine IM before a procedure to prevent nausea. The medication is available in a vial of 50 mg/mL. How many mL will you draw up in the syringe for this dose? _____ mL

4. A patient is to receive 0.5 mg of alprazolam PO. The medication is available in 1-mg tablets, which are scored. How many tablets will the patient receive? _____ tablet(s)

5. A patient is to receive 25 g of lactulose PO. The medication is a syrup that comes in unit dose packs of 10 g/15 mL. How much lactulose will you measure for the 25-g dose? _____ mL

6. A medication order reads "Give 200 mg of allopurinol PO daily." The medication is available in 100-mg tablets. Use the proportion method to calculate how many tablets the patient should receive. _____ tablet(s)

7. What happens to a drug dose calculation if you move the decimal point in error to the right?

8. What happens to a drug dose calculation if you move the decimal point in error to the left?

PRACTICE QUIZ

____ 1. In the formula $X = 45/90$, which element of the formula represents the numerator?
A. X
B. /
C. 45
D. 90

____ 2. Of the fractions listed below, which represents an improper fraction?
A. $\frac{1}{2}$
B. $1\frac{3}{4}$
C. $\frac{70}{35}$
D. $\frac{20}{100}$

____ 3. Which fraction correctly represents the whole number 55?
A. $\frac{55}{1}$
B. $\frac{1}{55}$
C. $\frac{55}{100}$
D. $\frac{5.5}{1}$

____ 4. Which fraction correctly represents $6\frac{7}{8}$?
A. $\frac{13}{8}$
B. $\frac{14}{7}$
C. $\frac{55}{8}$
D. $\frac{7}{14}$

____ 5. Which fraction is reduced to its lowest terms?
A. $\frac{3}{9}$
B. $\frac{5}{15}$
C. $\frac{6}{72}$
D. $\frac{4}{25}$

____ 6. What is the lowest common denominator for this series of fractions: $\frac{6}{8}$, $\frac{1}{3}$, $\frac{1}{2}$?
A. 8
B. 16
C. 24
D. 48

7. Calculate the answer to this problem: $\frac{6}{8} - \frac{3}{5}$. Reduce the fraction to its lowest terms.

8. Calculate the answer to this problem: $\frac{4}{12} \times \frac{1}{16}$. Reduce the fraction to its lowest terms.

9. Calculate the answer to this problem: $\frac{2}{3} \div \frac{5}{7}$. Reduce the fraction to its lowest terms.

____ 10. In the equation $3.33 \div 2.25 = 1.48$, which element is the dividend?
A. 3.33
B. 2.25
C. 1.48
D. =

11. Calculate the answer to this problem: 11.4×12.6, rounded to tenths.

12. Calculate the answer to this problem: $7.17 \div 11.16$, rounded to tenths.

____ 13. Which number expresses the fraction $\frac{3}{4}$ as a decimal?
A. 0.34
B. 3.4
C. .75
D. 0.75

____ 14. Which number expresses the decimal 6.3 as a fraction?
A. $\frac{2}{1}$
B. $\frac{6}{3}$
C. $6\frac{3}{10}$
D. $\frac{63}{1}$

____ 15. How much is 15% of 45?
A. 0.675
B. 6.75
C. 67.5
D. 675

16. The medication order reads "Nadolol, 180 mg, PO daily." The scored tablets are 120 mg/tablet. How many tablets will be given for this dose? _____ tablet(s)

17. The medication order reads "Megestrol, 120 mg, PO twice a day." The medication is available in unit-dose containers of 40 mg/mL. How much will be measured for each dose? _____ mL

18. The medication order reads "Furosemide, 80 mg, PO now." The medication is available in scored 40-mg tablets. Using the proportion method, calculate how many tablets will be given for this dose. _____ tablet(s)

Medical Systems of Weights and Measures

chapter

4

LEARNING ACTIVITIES

Matching

Match each definition with its corresponding term. (Not all terms will be used.)

_____ 1. A system of volume and weight measurements formerly used by physicians and pharmacists

_____ 2. Equal in amount or to have equal value

_____ 3. System of temperature measurement in which the freezing point of water is 32° above 0°

_____ 4. The basic metric unit for measurement of weight

_____ 5. The basic metric unit for measurement of length

_____ 6. System of temperature measurement in which the freezing point of water is 0°

A. Dimensional analysis
B. Equivalent
C. Celsius/centigrade
D. Gram
E. Liter
F. Apothecary
G. Fahrenheit
H. Meter

Fill in the Blank: Equivalents

Complete the following equivalents.

7. 1 pound = _____ ounces

8. _____ teaspoons = 1 tablespoon

9. 1 cup = _____ ounces

10. 1 gallon = _____ quarts

11. _____ feet = 1 yard

12. 32° F = _____ ° C

13. 1 kilogram = _____ grams

14. 1 gram = _____ milligrams

15. 1 liter = _____ milliliters

16. 1 centimeter = _____ millimeters

17. _____ pounds = 1 kilogram

18. 1 teaspoon = _____ milliliter(s)

19. _____ drops = 1 milliliter

20. 15 milliliters = _____ tablespoon(s)

21. 1 fluid ounce = _____ milliliter(s)

Fill in the Blank: Prefixes

For each prefix list the correct unit of measure and its abbreviation.

22. "kilo"   Weight: _____   Length: _____

23. "micro"   Weight: _____

24. "deci"   Liquids: _____

25. "centi"   Length: _____

26. "milli"   Weight: _____   Liquids: _____   Length: _____

27. "nano"   Weight: _____

MEDICATION SAFETY PRACTICE

State whether each statement is True or False. If the statement is false, rewrite it to make it true.

_____ 1. A liquid ounce is equal to a dry ounce.

_____ 2. Patients may use teaspoons and tablespoons from tableware to measure liquid drugs.

_____ 3. When measuring liquid drugs in a medicine cup, fill while holding the cup at eye level.

_____ 4. A 1-milligram tablet of a drug is 1000 times stronger than a 1-microgram tablet of that same drug.

_____ 5. A person's weight in kilograms is approximately double his or her weight in pounds.

_____ 6. The abbreviation "U" is acceptable for abbreviating "units" when dosing heparin.

_____ 7. Milliequivalents are used to measure electrolytes.

_____ 8. Insulin syringes may be interchanged with noninsulin syringes.

_____ 9. Normal human body temperature in Celsius/centigrade ranges between 36.1° and 37.8° C.

_____ 10. When giving liquid medication with a dropper, place the dropper into the side of the patient's mouth rather than in the middle where it can cause choking if it runs down the throat too quickly.

Conversions

Solve the following conversion problems, dosage problems, and drug calculations.

11. 100° F = _____ ° C

12. 39.5° C = _____ ° F

13. A patient is to take 2 tsp of cough syrup every 4 hours as needed for a cough. Convert 2 tsp to mL. _____ mL

14. 600 mL = _____ L

15. 2.5 L = _____ mL

16. 223 lbs = _____ kg

17. 79 kg = _____ lbs

18. 15 oz = _____ g

19. A patient is to receive a bolus injection of 8000 units of heparin. The vial of heparin contains 10,000 units/mL. How many milliliters will be drawn up into the syringe? _____ mL

PRACTICE QUIZ

_____ 1. Which unit is the basic measure of weight in the metric system?
   A. Dram
   B. Gram
   C. Meter
   D. Liter

2. Which statements about metric measurements are correct? (*Select all that apply.*)
   _____ A. A kilogram is 1000 times heavier than a gram.
   _____ B. A centimeter is 1/10 of a meter.
   _____ C. A milligram is 1000 times smaller than a gram.
   _____ D. A milliliter is 1/1000 of a liter.
   _____ E. A microgram is 1000 times heavier than a milligram.

_____ 3. An order for a liquid medication states to give "1 fluid ounce" per dose. The patient has a medication measuring device that is marked in tablespoons only. The patient is instructed that the dose of 1 fluid ounce equals how many tablespoons?
   A. ½
   B. 1
   C. 2
   D. 3

4. Which units are appropriate measures for solids? (*Select all that apply.*)
   _____ A. Ounce
   _____ B. Teaspoon
   _____ C. Drop
   _____ D. Gram
   _____ E. Milliliter
   _____ F. Nanogram

_____ 5. During an admission assessment, the patient weighs 109.1 kg. The patient asks the nurse, "What does that mean in pounds?" Which answer is correct?
   A. "You weigh 109.1 pounds."
   B. "You weigh 218 pounds."
   C. "You weigh 240 pounds."
   D. "You weigh 272.8 pounds."

6. A patient reports constipation and there is an order to give magnesium hydroxide, 1.5 ounces, at bedtime as needed. How many mL will be given to the patient? _____ mL

7. As part of a bowel preparation before a colonoscopy, a patient will need to take 15 doses of 200 mL of polyethylene glycol electrolyte solution every 10 minutes. After this prep is completed, how many liters of medication will the patient have consumed? _____ L

8. A patient will be receiving an intravenous dose of penicillin G potassium, 500,000 units per dose, every 6 hours. The medication is available in vials of 1 million units/50 mL. How many mL will the nurse draw up in the syringe to prepare an IV piggyback solution that contains 500,000 units of this medication? _____ mL

9. The nurse is preparing to administer a 10-mEq dose of oral potassium chloride liquid medication. The medication comes in unit dose packets of 20 mEq/15 mL. How many mL will the patient receive per dose? _____ mL

_____ 10. Digoxin 250 micrograms PO is prescribed. The medication is available in scored tablets of 0.25 mg each. How many tablets should be given to the patient?
   A. ⅒
   B. 1/25
   C. 1
   D. 10

Dosage Calculation of Intravenous Solutions and Drugs

chapter

5

LEARNING ACTIVITIES

Matching: Terminology Review

Match each definition with its corresponding term. (Use each term only once; not all terms will be used.)

_____ 1. How long (in minutes or hours) an IV infusion is ordered to run

_____ 2. Number of drops per minute needed to make an IV solution infuse in the prescribed amount of time

_____ 3. Number of drops needed to make 1 mL of IV fluid

_____ 4. Number of mL delivered in 1 hour of an IV infusion

_____ 5. Result of an infusion of IV fluids that occurs at a much faster rate than was ordered, causing harm to the patient

_____ 6. Leakage of irritating IV fluids into tissue surrounding the vein, resulting in tissue damage

_____ 7. Leakage of IV fluids into tissue surrounding the vein, resulting in tissue swelling

_____ 8. IV pump abbreviation for the volume of fluid that has already infused

_____ 9. Computer-based machine that pushes fluid into the vein by slow pressure

_____ 10. Device that uses gravity to control the flow of an IV

A. Controller
B. IV infusion pump
C. Fluid overload
D. Extravasation
E. Infiltration
F. Flow rate
G. Duration
H. Drop factor
I. Drip rate
J. VTBI
K. VI

Identification: IV Tubing Sets

For each tubing drop factor listed below, indicate whether the tubing that should be used is macrodrip or microdrip.

_____ 11. 10 drops/mL

_____ 12. 15 drops/mL

_____ 13. 20 drops/mL

_____ 14. 60 drops/mL

_____ 15. Used most often for children, older patients, and patients who cannot tolerate a fast infusion or a high volume of fluids

_____ 16. Used most often when fast infusion rates or larger quantities of fluids or drugs are needed

MEDICATION SAFETY PRACTICE

1. What term is used to indicate the time when the IV bag is supposed to be empty?

2. Safe or not safe: An IV infusion was supposed to be completed by 8 AM. It is now 9 AM and there is still 150 mL left in the IV bag. The infusion rate is increased in order to make up for lost time.

3. A drug order reads "Infuse 1000 mL of normal saline IV over 12 hours." Calculate the number of milliliters to be infused in 1 hour, based on this order.

4. Using the macrodrip formula, calculate the drip rate for this IV infusion order: "Infuse D_5W 1000 mL over 10 hours." The tubing's drop factor is 10.

5. Calculate the drip rate for this IV infusion order: "Infuse $D_5\frac{1}{2}NS$ at 50 mL/hour." The tubing's drop factor is 60.

6. Using the macrodrip tubing shortcut, calculate the drops per minute for this IV infusion order using tubing with a drop factor of 15: "Infuse NS at 75 mL/hour for 24 hours."

PRACTICE QUIZ

____ 1. A patient is very restless while receiving IV fluids to treat dehydration. The IV catheter has slipped out of the vein and fluid is delivered to the surrounding tissues under the skin, causing swelling. Which term best describes this occurrence?
   A. Infection
   B. Fluid overload
   C. Infiltration
   D. Extravasation

____ 2. Which IV tubing set delivers the smallest drops?
   A. 10 drops/mL
   B. 15 drops/mL
   C. 20 drops/mL
   D. 60 drops/mL

3. Which components are required for an order for IV fluids? *(Select all that apply.)*
   ____ A. Type of fluid to be administered
   ____ B. Controller device
   ____ C. Volume to be administered
   ____ D. Duration of fluid administration
   ____ E. Rate of fluid administration

4. An IV order reads "Infuse 2000 mL of normal saline over 24 hours." With a tubing set drop factor of 10, what is the drip rate for this IV infusion? _____ gtts/min

____ 5. A patient received an intravenous solution that led to tissue damage. What is the term used to describe this?
   A. Infiltration
   B. Extravasation
   C. Fluid overload
   D. IV pump failure

6. Using the "15-second" rule, calculate the drip rate for an IV infusion of 150 mL/hour. The tubing has a drip factor of 20. _____ gtts/min

7. An IV is to infuse at 36 drops per minute. How many drops should be counted in 15 seconds? _____ gtts in 15 seconds

____ 8. A patient is to receive intravenous fluids at a rate of 100 mL/hr. When the IV pump is programmed, a rate of 150 mL/hr is set. What will most likely occur?
   A. The computer will recognize the error and ignore the setting.
   B. An insufficient amount of fluids will be infused.
   C. The pump will alert the nurse to the error in the setting
   D. The pump will infuse the fluid at the settings as programmed.

____ 9. The following order was entered into the medical record of Howard P., age 78, who is receiving intravenous fluids to treat dehydration resulting from gastroenteritis. "Intravenous fluids at 125 mL/hr for 48 hours." The prescriber is contacted regarding which missing aspect of the order?
   A. Rate of infusion
   B. Volume to be infused
   C. Duration of treatment
   D. Type of fluids to be infused

____ 10. Which common IV pump setting prevents patients from tampering with the IV rate setting?
   A. STOP
   B. OFF switch
   C. Delete
   D. IV lock

11. A patient is to receive amphotericin B, which has been mixed in a 500-mL bag of IV fluid, over 5 hours. What is the flow rate for this infusion? _____ mL/hr

____ 12. A patient with gastroenteritis and dehydration has the following IV order: "1000 mL to infuse IV over 8 hours." Microdrip tubing is available. What is the nurse's best action?
   A. Ask the prescriber to clarify the rate in drops per minute.
   B. Administer the IV fluids at 125 drops per minute.
   C. Ask the prescriber to clarify the type of fluid to be infused.
   D. Administer the IV fluid using a controller device at 125 mL/hour.

Anti-Inflammatory Drugs

LEARNING ACTIVITIES

Identification: Infection or Inflammation?

For the following, place an X in the column (A or B) that matches the characteristics of each, infection and inflammation.

	A: Infection	B: Inflammation
1. Normal reaction of the body to injury or invasion		
2. Invasion of the body by microorganisms		
3. Allergic reactions (hayfever, asthma)		
4. Nonspecific (same tissue response for any location or cause)		
5. Manifests with sprained joints and blisters		
6. Disturbs the normal environment and causes harm		

Multiple Response

7. Which are common side effects or adverse effects of corticosteroids?
   (Select all that apply.)
   ____ A. Sodium and fluid loss
   ____ B. Hypertension
   ____ C. Excessive sleeping
   ____ D. Nervousness
   ____ E. Weight loss
   ____ F. Moon face
   ____ G. Buffalo hump
   ____ H. Fragile skin
   ____ I. Excessive muscle strength
   ____ J. Thickened scalp hair

8. Which are signs and symptoms of acute adrenal insufficiency? *(Select all that apply.)*
   ____ A. Confusion
   ____ B. Muscle weakness
   ____ C. Rapid irregular pulse
   ____ D. Nausea and vomiting
   ____ E. Salt craving
   ____ F. Weight loss

Matching

Match each term with its corresponding definition. (Use each term only once; not all terms will be used.)

_____ 9. Antihistamines

_____ 10. Anti-inflammatory drugs

_____ 11. Corticosteroids

_____ 12. Disease-modifying antirheumatic drugs (DMARDs)

_____ 13. Nonsteroidal anti-inflammatory drugs (NSAIDs)

A. Prevent or limit inflammation by slowing or stopping inflammatory mediator production

B. A chemical that binds to receptor sites and causes inflammatory responses

C. Prevent or limit the tissue and blood vessel responses to injury or invasion by slowing the production of one or more inflammatory mediators

D. Reduces the progression and tissue destruction of the inflammatory disease process by inhibiting tumor necrosis factor

E. Prevents inflammatory mediator histamine from binding to its receptor site

F. Drugs that prevent or limit inflammatory responses to injury or invasion

Matching: Inflammatory Response

Match the characteristics associated with stages I, II, or III of the inflammatory response. (Answers may be used more than once.)

_____ 14. Lasts until healing is complete.

_____ 15. Mediators are released that make blood vessels dilate and become leaky.

_____ 16. Characterized by redness, swelling, and pain.

_____ 17. Begins at the initial injury but may not be evident until the exudate stage is over.

_____ 18. Characterized by increased secretions.

_____ 19. May be accompanied by a low-grade fever.

_____ 20. Known as the stage of tissue repair.

_____ 21. Many new cells come to the area and release more mediators.

_____ 22. Known as the exudate stage.

_____ 23. Begins within minutes after the injury or invasion and lasts for hours.

_____ 24. Cells are stimulated to divide and form scar tissue.

_____ 25. Known as the vascular stage.

A. Stage I

B. Stage II

C. Stage III

Matching: Nonsteroidal Anti-Inflammatory Drugs

Match the trade or brand names of the following NSAIDs with their corresponding generic names. (Drug names may be used more than once.)

_____ 26. Ibuprofen
_____ 27. Naproxen
_____ 28. Celecoxib
_____ 29. Oxaprozin
_____ 30. Aspirin
_____ 31. Piroxicam
_____ 32. Indomethacin
_____ 33. Meclofenamic acid
_____ 34. Mefenamic acid
_____ 35. Ketorolac

A. Indocin
B. Motrin
C. Ecotrin
D. Ponstel
E. Toradol
F. Celebrex
G. Naprosyn
H. Aleve
I. Meclomen
J. Daypro
K. Feldene
L. Advil

Fill in the Blank

36. During stage _____ of the inflammatory response, large numbers of white blood cells are created.

37. Exudate (tissue drainage) is also commonly referred to as _____.

38. Loss of function can occur when damaged tissues are replaced with _____ tissue.

39. A patient who is to receive instructions on use of adalimumab (Humira) should be taught how to give an injection by the _____ route.

40. A patient with severe _____ _____ should not receive DMARDs.

MEDICATION SAFETY PRACTICE

1. All of the NSAIDs except aspirin can reduce blood flow to which organ? _____

2. Which is the only NSAID recommended for children? _____

3. Compared to the recommended adult dose of cetirizine (Zyrtec), the common dose for children is _____.

4. A child weighing 35 pounds has an IM injection of methylprednisolone (Solu-Medrol) 30 mg prescribed. Does this fall within the recommended range? Why or why not?

5. A patient is to receive prednisone 10 mg PO at 8 AM. The medication tray is supplied with prednisolone 20-mg scored tablets. What action should be taken?

6. Several patients will be receiving an initial injection of a DMARD in the clinic today. What safety precautions should be in place? What is a common problem with the site of injection of a DMARD?

PRACTICE QUIZ

_____ 1. A community health educator is discussing aspirin use. Which instruction is most appropriate regarding aspirin use in children?
   A. It is frequently used to prevent febrile seizures in children with influenza.
   B. It is contraindicated in children due to the risk of developing Reye's syndrome.
   C. It is recommended to treat fever and discomfort caused by chickenpox.
   D. It is associated with Reye's syndrome, a form of renal failure.

2. Which are common assessment findings for a patient who has used corticosteroids for several months? _(Select all that apply.)_
   _____ A. Decreased facial hair
   _____ B. Decreased waist circumference
   _____ C. Increased fat distribution between shoulders
   _____ D. Muscle wasting
   _____ E. Abdominal striae

_____ 3. A patient taking corticosteroids should have which instruction included in patient teaching to avoid stomach ulcers?
   A. Take the medication just before bedtime.
   B. Take the medication by injection.
   C. Take the medication on an empty stomach.
   D. Take the medication with food.

_____ 4. Male patients should be instructed to use antihistamines with caution due to the risk of which side effect?
   A. Confusion
   B. Hypertension
   C. Urinary retention
   D. Nausea

_____ 5. A patient who is taking an antihistamine that causes drowsiness must be taught that additional drowsiness may result if the medication is combined with which element?
   A. Carbohydrate-rich meal
   B. Green leafy vegetables
   C. Alcoholic beverages
   D. Grapefruit juice

_____ 6. An older adult patient who is on corticosteroids for severe arthritis is looking forward to a visit from her preschool-aged grandchildren. The priority instructions that should be given to this patient should include information that she is at a higher risk for which condition?
A. Infection
B. Muscle atrophy
C. Weight changes
D. Nausea and vomiting

_____ 7. A patient with diabetes is prescribed corticosteroids for asthma. This patient will require additional monitoring for which condition?
A. Abdominal striae
B. Weight loss
C. Increased blood glucose
D. Fluid retention

_____ 8. A patient with a sprained ankle asks why the ankle is swollen. On what knowledge is the nurse's response based?
A. Infection is occurring in the injured area.
B. Blood vessel constriction is causing the swelling.
C. Capillaries leak fluid into the tissues.
D. Slowed white blood cell production causes the swelling.

_____ 9. A patient taking 50 mg of celecoxib (Celebrex) for arthritis pain should be instructed to immediately report which occurrence to the prescriber?
A. Bruising
B. Gum bleeding
C. Anorexia
D. Chest pain

_____ 10. A patient who is taking a COX-1 NSAID is scheduled for surgery in a week. What is the patient at increased risk for?
A. Bleeding
B. Infection
C. Nausea
D. Deep vein thrombosis

_____ 11. The nurse will be administering a daily NSAID to a patient. When is the best time to administer this medication?
A. Between meals
B. Any time
C. With meals or milk
D. At bedtime

_____ 12. A patient taking a leukotriene inhibitor should be monitored for which common side effect?
A. Headache
B. Hives
C. Liver impairment
D. Anaphylaxis

Drugs for Pain Control

chapter
7

LEARNING ACTIVITIES

Crossword Puzzle: Terminology Review

Complete the puzzle by identifying the key terms that are described.

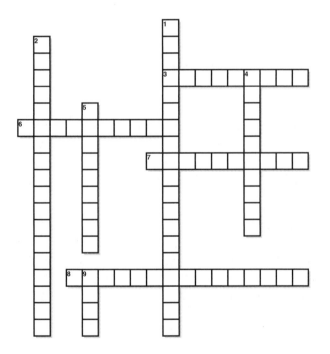

Across

3. The adjustment of the body to long-term opioid use that increases the elimination rate of the drug and reduces the main effects (pain relief) and side effects of the drug
6. Autonomic nervous system symptoms occurring when long-term opioid therapy is stopped suddenly after physical dependence is present
7. Physical changes in autonomic nervous system function that can occur when opioids are used long-term and are not needed for pain control
8. A drug containing any ingredient derived from the poppy plant (or a similar synthetic chemical) that changes a person's perception of pain and has a potential for psychological or physical dependence (two words)

Down

1. A drug containing ingredients known to be addictive that is regulated by the Federal Controlled Substances Act of 1970 (two words)
2. A drug that reduces a person's perception of pain; it is not similar to opium and has little potential for psychological or physical dependence (two words)
4. Drugs of any class that provide pain relief either by changing the perception of pain or by reducing its source
5. The psychologic need or craving for the "high" feeling that results from using opioids when pain is not present
9. An unpleasant sensory and emotional experience associated with acute or potential tissue damage; pain is whatever a patient says it is and exists whenever a patient says it does

Matching

Match the statements about types of pain on the left with the terms on the right. (Not all terms will be used.)

_____ 1. Physical changes in the autonomic nervous system function that can occur when opioids are used long-term and are not needed for pain control.

_____ 2. The psychological need or craving for the "high" feeling that results from using opioids when pain is not present

_____ 3. The point at which pain is perceived

_____ 4. The adjustment of the body to long-term opioid use that reduces the pain relief of the drug

_____ 5. Autonomic nervous system symptoms occurring when long-term opioid therapy is stopped suddenly after physical dependence is present

A. Tolerance
B. Addiction
C. Dependence
D. Withdrawal
E. Pain threshold
F. Pain tolerance

Identification: Types of Pain

For each pain characteristic listed, label as "A" for acute pain or "C" for chronic pain.

_____ 6. Often has an identifiable cause

_____ 7. Exact cause may or may not be known

_____ 8. Pain may be described as burning, aching, or throbbing

_____ 9. Pain may be described as sharp, stabbing, or pricking

_____ 10. Improves with time

_____ 11. Does not improve with time, and may even worsen

_____ 12. Unlimited duration

_____ 13. Limited duration

_____ 14. Triggers physiologic responses such as increased heart rate and breathing

_____ 15. Physiologic responses go away over time

MEDICATION SAFETY PRACTICE

For each statement below, label the drug as Schedule I, II, III, or IV, and provide one example of a drug in that schedule.

_____ 1. Accepted for medical use in the U.S., and has a low potential for abuse compared to drugs in other schedules.

_____ 2. A high potential for abuse, but is accepted for use as a treatment in the U.S. However, abuse may lead to severe psychological or physical dependence.

_____ 3. Currently accepted for treatment in the U.S., and the potential for abuse is lower than most of the drugs in other schedules. However, abuse may lead to moderate or low physical dependence or high psychological dependence.

_____ 4. The lowest potential for abuse compared to drugs in other schedules, and may be found in cough and antidiarrheal preparations.

_____ 5. Not accepted for medical use in treatment in the U.S., and has a high potential for abuse.

Briefly answer each question after reading the scenario below.

Mr. B. has been prescribed morphine for postoperative pain control. He calls the nurse to ask for pain medication, and states that his pain rating is at "8." His last dose of pain medication was 6 hours ago.

6. Before administering the drug, what two assessment parameters are most important to assess?

7. Mr. B. states, "That pain medicine really knocks me out! But it sure helps with the pain." What information is most important to teach the patient at this time?

8. The medication order reads, "morphine, oral solution (Roxanol), 15 mg every 4 hours, PO, as needed for pain." The medication is available in a unit-dose solution of 10 mg/5 mL. How many mL will be administered for the ordered dose? _____ mL

PRACTICE QUIZ

1. Which factors may reduce a patient's pain tolerance? _(Select all that apply.)_
   _____ A. Fear
   _____ B. Distraction
   _____ C. Lack of sleep
   _____ D. Relaxation
   _____ E. Anxiety

_____ 2. A patient who is experiencing chronic pain would likely experience which symptoms?
   A. Burning, aching, or throbbing pain
   B. Pain felt superficially on the body
   C. Increased heart rate and blood pressure
   D. Sweating and increased respiratory rate

3. A patient will be receiving extra-strength acetaminophen (Tylenol) for pain following hernia surgery. Which conditions may be of concern if found in the patient's history? *(Select all that apply.)*
   - ____ A. Liver disease
   - ____ B. History of alcoholism
   - ____ C. Arthritis
   - ____ D. Hypothyroidism
   - ____ E. Kidney disease

____ 4. A patient states, "I've had this pain for almost a year and my doctor told me I need to take an antidepressant. What's that for? I'm not depressed!" Which answer is most appropriate?
   - A. "Maybe you really are depressed and just not aware of it."
   - B. "Your doctor is concerned you might be addicted to pain medication."
   - C. "Antidepressants help increase the amount of endorphins in the brain."
   - D. "You have likely developed a tolerance to effects of pain medications."

____ 5. A patient is receiving an opioid drug through patient-controlled analgesia. Which patient assessment finding, if noted, is of most concern?
   - A. A sleeping patient who wakes up when called by name
   - B. Reports of nausea
   - C. Respiratory rate of 8 breaths per minute
   - D. Oxygenation saturation of 96% on room air

____ 6. A patient reports feeling nauseated after taking an oral opioid for pain. Which action is most appropriate?
   - A. Instruct the patient to take the medication with food.
   - B. Tell the patient that the nausea will pass after a few doses.
   - C. Ask the prescriber to order the opioid in an intravenous form.
   - D. Provide the patient with a low-fiber diet.

____ 7. A 5-year-old child reports pain after a tonsillectomy, saying "My throat really hurts." The child is to receive opioids. When medicating this patient, which intervention is most appropriate?
   - A. Use the FLACC scale to determine the child's relative pain intensity.
   - B. Recognize that many surgical procedures are not as painful for children as for adults.
   - C. Observe for the common side effect of diarrhea, and administer antidiarrheals as needed.
   - D. Use an apnea monitor, pulse oximetry, and frequent assessments after medicating the child.

____ 8. A patient has ingested a large amount of acetaminophen. Which medication will need to be administered to prevent liver damage?
   - A. Acetylcysteine
   - B. Naloxone
   - C. Naltrexone
   - D. Hydromorphone

____ 9. A patient has received a parenteral dose of hydromorphone. Thirty minutes later, the patient's respiratory rate is 8 breaths per minute, and the patient is extremely drowsy. Which action should occur first?
   - A. Assess the patient's blood pressure.
   - B. Gently shake the patient's arm.
   - C. Squeeze the patient's trapezius muscle.
   - D. Apply firm pressure to the nail bed.

____ 10. A patient is taking an extended-release (ER) dose of hydrocodone to treat cancer pain. The patient is advised to change positions slowly to avoid which common side effect?
   - A. Drug tolerance
   - B. Respiratory depression
   - C. Hallucinations
   - D. Orthostatic hypotension

____ 11. A patient with chronic pain has difficulty swallowing tablets and capsules and would also like to avoid injections for as long as possible. Which drug is available as a lollipop?
   A. Oxycodone
   B. Tramadol
   C. Fentanyl
   D. Meperidine

12. Which interventions are appropriate to take after administering an opioid drug to a patient who has sustained a fractured humerus? *(Select all that apply.)*
   ____ A. If the patient's respiratory rate is 14/min, awaken the patient by calling his or her name.
   ____ B. Warn the patient that pupil dilation is common while taking this category of drugs.
   ____ C. Have naloxone (Narcan) available in the emergency cart in the event a reversal is needed.
   ____ D. Remind the patient to call for help before getting out of bed to ambulate.
   ____ E. Place side rails up and the call light within easy reach of the patient.

____ 13. Which drug is most likely prescribed to treat a patient's pain and burning from diabetic neuropathy?
   A. Acetaminophen (Tylenol)
   B. Pregabalin (Lyrica)
   C. Ibuprofen (Motrin, Advil)
   D. Oxycodone (Percodan)

____ 14. All of these medications are in the narcotics storage unit. Which one has the highest potential for abuse?
   A. Fentanyl
   B. Tylenol No. 4
   C. tramadol (Ultram)
   D. Cough syrup with codeine

Anti-Infectives: Antibacterial Drugs

LEARNING ACTIVITIES

Identification: Drug Categories

Identify the drug category described.

1. Kills susceptible bacteria by preventing them from forming strong protective cell walls.

    _____

2. Enters bacterial cells and prevents bacteria reproduction by suppressing the actions of enzymes important in making bacterial DNA.

    _____

3. Interferes with bacterial reproduction by preventing the bacteria from making proteins important to their life cycles and infective processes.

    _____

4. Prevents bacteria from making proteins important to their life cycles and infective processes.

    _____

Matching

Match the terms on the right with the descriptions on the left. (Not all descriptions will be used.)

____ 5.   Ability of bacteria to invade and spread

____ 6.   Also known as "blood poisoning"

____ 7.   Single-celled organisms that have their own DNA

____ 8.   Drug that kills bacteria directly

____ 9.   Organism that causes infection when the immune system is suppressed

____ 10. Most common cause of death worldwide

____ 11. Organism that does not cause infection or systemic disease

____ 12. Drug that prevents bacteria from dividing and growing

A. Nonpathogenic
B. Bactericidal
C. Infection
D. Bacteriostatic
E. Bacteria
F. Opportunistic organism
G. Sepsis
H. Virulence

Matching: Cell Wall Synthesis Inhibitors

Match the trade or brand names of the following cell wall synthesis inhibitor drugs with their corresponding generic names. (Use each term only once.)

_____ 13. Amoxil

_____ 14. Ancef

_____ 15. Azactam

_____ 16. Bicillin LA

_____ 17. Invanz

_____ 18. Keflex

_____ 19. Merrem

_____ 20. Rocephin

_____ 21. Timentin

_____ 22. Vancocin

A. cephalexin
B. ceftriaxone
C. vancomycin
D. aztreonam
E. ticarcillin/clavulanate
F. amoxicillin
G. meropenem
H. penicillin G benzathine
I. ertapenem
J. cefazolin

Matching: Protein Synthesis Inhibitors

Match the protein synthesis inhibitor drugs to their corresponding use, action, side effect, precaution, or adverse effect. (Use each term only once.)

_____ 23. A parenteral drug that can seriously reduce hearing

_____ 24. Usually prescribed for infections of the skin and respiratory tract in people who are allergic to penicillins and cephalosporins

_____ 25. Can cause significant joint and muscle pain

_____ 26. Enhances the effect of warfarin and greatly increases the risk for bleeding in patients taking both drugs

_____ 27. Can cause severe respiratory depression in infants and children

_____ 28. Has no effect on bacteria that do not require oxygen for survival or metabolism

_____ 29. An oral drug used to treat MRSA

_____ 30. Can cause a permanent gray-yellow staining to tooth enamel if taken during tooth development

A. tetracycline
B. linezolid
C. dalfopristin
D. azithromycin
E. amikacin
F. clarithromycin
G. streptomycin
H. macrolides

Matching: Sulfonamides/Trimethoprim, Fluoroquinolones

Match the actions, uses, side effects, precautions, and adverse effects associated with sulfonamides/trimethoprim and fluoroquinolones. (Terms may be used more than once.)

_____ 31. Tendon rupture

_____ 32. Used to treat and prevent anthrax

_____ 33. Prevent(s) conversion of substances into folic acid

_____ 34. Bactericidal rather than bacteriostatic

_____ 35. Can form crystals in the kidney

_____ 36. Concentrate in urine, causing irritation of nearby tissues

_____ 37. Should not be given to anyone who has a G6PD deficiency

_____ 38. Avoided in infants because severe jaundice is likely to result

_____ 39. Avoided in infants and children because of potential damage to muscle and bone

_____ 40. Used to treat pneumocystis pneumonia

_____ 41. Can cause noninfectious hepatitis

_____ 42. Is associated with a cardiac problem known as "long QT syndrome"

A. Fluoroquinolones
B. Sulfonamides/ trimethoprim

Identification: Bacteria

Identify the type of bacteria described.

43. Bacteria that cause infection. _____

44. Nonpathogenic bacteria always present on skin and mucous membranes and in the GI tract.

_____

45. Bacteria that cause disease only in someone whose immune system is not working well.

_____

MEDICATION SAFETY PRACTICE

1. A child weighing 22 pounds is prescribed amoxicillin/clavulanic acid (Augmentin) for otitis media. What is the correct dosage to administer every 8 hours? _____

2. A patient who is allergic to penicillin may also be allergic to

_____ .

3. A 7-year-old child with a urinary tract infection is prescribed oral trimethoprim/sulfamethoxazole (Bactrim) to take orally. The child weighs 44 pounds. The recommended children's dose based on trimethoprim content is 3-6 mg/kg orally every 12 hours. What is the correct dose for this patient?

_____

4. List three signs and symptoms of an anaphylactic drug reaction.

_____

_____

_____

5. A patient is taking a sulfonamide drug and has been advised to increase oral fluids. What is the reason these instructions are given?

_____

_____

PRACTICE QUIZ

_____ 1. A patient has been prescribed imipenem/cilastatin (Primaxin). Which is a potential adverse effect of this drug?
  A. Unplanned pregnancy
  B. Interaction with asthma medication
  C. Seizures
  D. "Red man" syndrome

_____ 2. Which serious adverse effect could occur with vancomycin (Vancocin)?
  A. Reduced kidney function
  B. Impaired liver function
  C. Decreased white blood cell production
  D. Impaired clotting ability

_____ 3. A patient is receiving an IV piggyback containing ticarcillin/clavulanic acid (Timentin) and develops difficulty breathing and swelling of the mouth and throat. What is the first action to take?
  A. Remove the IV access device.
  B. Notify the prescriber.
  C. Determine the patient's allergies.
  D. Stop the infusion of the drug.

_____ 4. An older adult is prescribed gentamicin. Which assessments are most appropriate to make? (Select all that apply.)
  _____ A. Intake and output
  _____ B. Appetite
  _____ C. Bowel elimination
  _____ D. Hearing ability
  _____ E. Joint pain

_____ 5. A patient is taking the oral antibiotic cefdinir (Omnicef) to treat a skin wound infection. Which information is crucial to include in patient teaching?
  A. "This medication may also help your sore throat."
  B. "If bloody stools develop, contact your prescriber."
  C. "After your skin infection clears, stop taking the medication."
  D. "If a vaginal yeast infection occurs, discontinue using this medication."

_____ 6. Ciprofloxacin (Cipro) has been prescribed for a patient who is also taking an antacid. How should these medications be administered?
  A. Omit the prescribed antacid until the ciprofloxacin is no longer necessary.
  B. Administer ciprofloxacin 2 hours before giving the antacid.
  C. Administer ciprofloxacin 2 hours after giving the antacid.
  D. Omit the ciprofloxacin until antacids are no longer necessary.

_____ 7. A patient is taking both a macrolide antibacterial drug and warfarin (Coumadin). The patient should be instructed to observe closely for increased likelihood of which condition?
   A. Coronary thrombosis
   B. Cardiac dysrhythmias
   C. Excessive bleeding
   D. Antibiotic resistance

_____ 8. An older adult is taking levofloxacin (Levaquin) to treat a urinary tract infection. What is the best action to take if this patient develops new onset of pain and inflammation of the Achilles tendon of the heel?
   A. Administer prescribed PRN pain medication.
   B. Assist the patient in learning crutch walking.
   C. Ask the prescriber for a physical therapy consult.
   D. Notify the prescriber of an adverse effect.

_____ 9. Which patient assessment finding most closely indicates a serious adverse effect of trimethoprim/sulfamethoxazole (Bactrim)?
   A. Increased sun sensitivity
   B. Polycythemia
   C. Skin peeling, sloughing, and blisters
   D. Appearance of thrush in the mouth

_____ 10. A woman who is pregnant asks the nurse midwife to prescribe tetracyclines to treat facial acne. She asks why this medication cannot be used during pregnancy. Which is the best response?
   A. Tetracycline can cause a permanent discoloration of the teeth and thin tooth enamel.
   B. Tetracycline can cause damage to the tendons of the developing fetus during pregnancy.
   C. Tetracycline during pregnancy can be associated with allergic responses later in life.
   D. Tetracycline can be resumed once the baby is born, and the mother is breastfeeding.

Anti-Infectives: Antiviral Drugs

LEARNING ACTIVITIES

Identification: HAART

In the following list of drugs, indicate which might be included in an antiretroviral HAART regimen (H), and which would not (NonH).

_____ 1.   abacavir (Ziagen)

_____ 2.   acyclovir (Zovirax)

_____ 3.   amantadine (Symmetrel)

_____ 4.   didanosine (ddI, Videx)

_____ 5.   zidovudine (Retrovir)

_____ 6.   valacyclovir (Valtrex)

_____ 7.   oseltamivir (Tamiflu)

_____ 8.   emtricitabine (Emtriva)

_____ 9.   zanamivir (Relenza)

Matching

Match the correct definition on the right with its term on the left. (Answers will be used only once.)

_____ 10. Teratogen

_____ 11. Retrovirus

_____ 12. Virulence

_____ 13. Virustatic

_____ 14. Viral load

_____ 15. Common virus

_____ 16. HIV

_____ 17. Opportunistic infection

A. Overgrowth of normally present organisms
B. Number of viral particles in a blood sample
C. Virus that can use either DNA or RNA as its genetic material
D. Organism that causes AIDS
E. An agent that can cause birth defects
F. Measure of how well an organism can invade and grow
G. A virus that uses RNA as its genetic material
H. Drug action that prevents viral growth and reproduction

Matching: Antiviral Drugs

Match each antiviral drug to its corresponding use, action, side effect, precaution, or adverse effect. (Use each term only once.)

_____ 18. Highly teratogenic

_____ 19. Administered by oral inhalation only

_____ 20. Dilute parenteral form only with sterile water for injection

_____ 21. Oral suspension requires specific preparation immediately before administration

_____ 22. Has fewer central nervous system side effects than amantadine

_____ 23. Is converted to acyclovir at the cellular level

_____ 24. Can be confused with Zyvox

_____ 25. Can be confused with Valcyte

A. Oseltamivir
B. Relenza
C. Virazole
D. Amantadine
E. Zovirax
F. Rimantadine
G. Valacyclovir
H. Valtrex

Matching: Antiretroviral Drugs

Match each antiretroviral drug or category to its corresponding use, action, side effect, precaution, or adverse effect. (Use each term only once.)

_____ 26. Prevents cellular infection by blocking the CCR5 receptor on CD4+ cells

_____ 27. Increase the risk for lactic acidosis in pregnant women

_____ 28. Can be confused with Viracept

_____ 29. Must be given with ritonavir to achieve a high enough blood level to be effective

_____ 30. Is most likely to cause hypersensitivity reactions within the first 4 weeks of therapy

_____ 31. Can only be administered by subcutaneous injection

_____ 32. Should not be administered to any person who is allergic to sulfa drugs

_____ 33. Should not be prescribed for pregnant women if the patient's viral load indicates that traditional HAART is effective

_____ 34. Generic names of drugs in this class usually have "vir" in the middle of the name

_____ 35. Can be confused with Retrovir

_____ 36. Patients should avoid taking St. John's wort with any drug from this class

_____ 37. Can be confused with lamotrigine

A. Viramune
B. abacavir
C. darunavir
D. ritonavir
E. NNRTIs
F. Prezista
G. NRTIs
H. maraviroc
I. enfuvirtide
J. raltegravir
K. protease inhibitors
L. lamivudine

Labeling

In the figure below, label the five parts of a common virus.

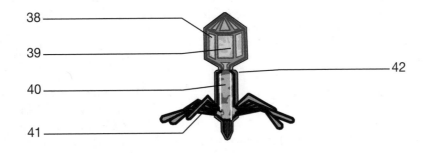

38 ———————
39 ———————
40 ———————
41 ———————
42

MEDICATION SAFETY PRACTICE

Fill in the Blank

Fill in the blanks with the correct answers.

1. The usual type of tissue through which viruses enter the body is

   _____ _____.

2. Following a regular schedule is critical in antiviral therapy in order to maintain an adequate _____ _____.

3. Before administering ribavirin (Virazole), the patient's _____ and _____ counts must be checked because of the risk for bone marrow suppression.

4. The correct dosage of abacavir (Ziagen) every 12 hours for a child who weighs 44 pounds (20 kg) is _____ mg.

5. Enfuvirtide (Fuzeon) which has not been mixed with water is stored between _____° and _____° F.

6. The risk of rhabdomyolysis in patients taking raltegravir (Isentress) is increased when taken with _____-type drugs.

PRACTICE QUIZ

_____ 1. A child weighing 66 pounds is to receive amantadine (Symmetrel) orally to treat influenza A. What is the correct dose to administer every 12 hours?
   A. 2.5 mg
   B. 30 mg
   C. 75 mg
   D. 100 mg

_____ 2. Before administering the first dose of valacyclovir (Valtrex) to a patient, you review the chart and note that the patient is also taking phenytoin (Dilantin) for a seizure disorder. The prescriber is notified because of which action of the antiviral drug?
   A. Lowering the seizure threshold
   B. Increasing the level of the drug in the blood
   C. Reducing the effectiveness of anticonvulsant drugs
   D. Causing nausea and vomiting

____ 3. A 70-year-old patient is taking rimantadine (Flumadine) for treatment of influenza. He calls the clinic to report that he
has gained 4 pounds over the weekend,
and his ankles are swollen. The patient
will need further evaluation for what condition?
   A. Lymphedema
   B. Pneumonia
   C. Heart failure
   D. Atrial fibrillation

____ 4. Administering ribavirin (Copegus) is con-
traindicated for any patient with which
condition?
   A. Influenza
   B. Pregnancy
   C. Seasonal allergies
   D. Open sores

____ 5. A diabetic patient on antiretroviral drugs
has a marked increase in fasting blood
glucose. Which intervention do you an-
ticipate from the prescriber?
   A. A decrease in dosage of the antiretroviral drug
   B. An increase in dosage of the antidiabetic drug
   C. Beginning administration of a different antidiabetic drug
   D. A decrease in the patient's carbohy-
drate intake

____ 6. To assess for liver function in patients
who are receiving antiretroviral drugs,
what should be done daily?
   A. Monitor the blood urea nitrogen
(BUN) level.
   B. Check stool color.
   C. Assess the sclera of the eyes.
   D. Measure intake and output.

____ 7. Which statement shows a patient's understanding of the administration schedule
of antiretroviral drugs?
   A. "I take the pills whenever I wake up
in the morning."
   B. "If I miss a dose, I don't worry about
it."
   C. "I have a printed schedule and I follow it closely every day."
   D. "When I miss a dose, I just double the
amount next time."

____ 8. Which intervention will be most useful
for a patient with peripheral neuropathy
as a side effect of antiretroviral drugs?
   A. Restricting fluid intake
   B. Avoiding apples, prunes, and bran
cereal
   C. Inspecting feet daily
   D. Wearing new shoes until broken in

____ 9. A 1-year-old child has been diagnosed
as being HIV-positive and has been prescribed a nonnucleoside analog reverse
transcriptase inhibitor (NNRTI) drug.
Which instruction is included in this patient's care?
   A. Children should not receive NNRTIs
until age 16.
   B. Give this medication with an antacid
to decrease nausea.
   C. Monitor for anemia by assessing for
pallor, fatigue, or cyanosis.
   D. If depression develops, St. John's
wort is frequently prescribed.

____ 10. A 27-year-old sexually active woman
is taking ribavirin (Copegus, Virazole).
Which plan for contraception is appropri-
ate for her?
   A. Oral contraception
   B. Condoms
   C. Intrauterine device
   D. Any combination of two methods

11. A patient has been prescribed acyclovir
(Zovirax) to treat varicella zoster. The
patient will be monitored for which com-
mon side effects of acyclovir? *(Select all
that apply.)*
   ____ A. Liver failure
   ____ B. Bone marrow suppression
   ____ C. Headache
   ____ D. Dizziness
   ____ E. Nausea

Anti-Infectives: Antitubercular and Antifungal Drugs

LEARNING ACTIVITIES

Matching

Match the possible side effect or adverse effect on the right with the drug listed on the left. (Each option will be used only once.)

_____ 1.   isoniazid (INH)

_____ 2.   rifampin (Rifadin, Rimactane)

_____ 3.   pyrazinamide (PZA)

_____ 4.   ethambutol (EMB, Myambutol)

A.   Optic neuritis
B.   Peripheral neuropathy
C.   Reddish-orange stain to secretions
D.   Increased uric acid formation

Fill in the Blank

5.   For ringworm of the scalp, children may be prescribed the drug _____.

6.   A patient who is taking isoniazid should avoid _____ to prevent hypertension.

7.   A patient's skin and urine may be stained _____ when taking rifampin.

8.   When taking a TB drug regimen, severe sunburn can be avoided by which measures?

9.   The risk for liver toxicity when taking first-line anti-TB drugs is higher in _____ populations.

10.   A patient taking terbinafine (Lamisil) has a reduced white blood cell count and is at higher risk for _____.

Matching: Types of Drugs for Tuberculosis

Match the characteristics, side effects, or precautions associated with the specific antitu-
berculosis drugs. (Drug names may be used more than once.)

_____ 11. Important for patients to see an ophthalmologist while taking
         this drug

_____ 12. Can raise blood pressure to dangerously high levels if taken
         with caffeine

_____ 13. Can cause breast tenderness in males

_____ 14. Teach patients that this drug colors the urine and other
         secretions a reddish-orange

_____ 15. Reduces the pH of intracellular fluid inside white blood cells
         that are infected with the TB bacillus

_____ 16. Can cause peripheral neuropathy, especially in patients who
         are malnourished

_____ 17. Should not be taken by infants and young children even when
         they have active tuberculosis

_____ 18. Is only bacteriostatic and must be used in combination with
         other antituberculosis drugs to be effective

_____ 19. Increases muscle aches and pains

_____ 20. Increased sensitivity to sun and ultraviolet light

_____ 21. May cause loss of appetite, difficulty concentrating, and sore
         throat

_____ 22. Pregnant women need higher doses of B-complex vitamins
         while taking this drug

A. ethambutol
B. isoniazid
C. pyrazinamide
D. rifampin

Matching: Antifungal Drugs

Match the trade or brand names of these antifungal drugs with their corresponding
generic names. (Use each term only once.)

_____ 23. Ancobon

_____ 24. Cancidas

_____ 25. Diflucan

_____ 26. Eraxis

_____ 27. Fungizone

_____ 28. Lamisil

_____ 29. Mycamine

_____ 30. Nizoral

_____ 31. Noxafil

_____ 32. Vfend

A. flucytosine
B. micafungin
C. caspofungin
D. fluconazole
E. terbinafine
F. ketoconazole
G. anidulafungin
H. amphotericin B
I. posaconazole
J. voriconazole

MEDICATION SAFETY PRACTICE

1. An older adult who is taking an echinocandin is at increased risk for developing deep vein thrombosis. Which interventions can help prevent this? *(Select all that apply.)*
    ____ A. Heparin drip
    ____ B. Venous sequential compression device
    ____ C. Deep tissue massage to legs
    ____ D. Range-of-motion exercises
    ____ E. Ambulation
    ____ F. Ace bandage wraps to legs
    ____ G. Adequate fluid intake

2. Based on a dosage formula of 4 mg/kg, the correct dose of ketoconazole (Extina, Nizoral) for a child who weighs 22 pounds is _____ mg.

3. The correct maximum daily dose for pyrazinamide (PZA) is _____ mg.

4. A patient says she stopped taking her medication to treat tuberculosis after a month, because she stopped coughing up blood. The patient should be instructed to continue taking the medication for how long?

    _____

5. A patient who is taking several first-line medications to treat tuberculosis says he likes to drink several cans of beer after work every night. He is advised to stop drinking to avoid developing which adverse effect?

    _____

PRACTICE QUIZ

1. High doses of ethambutol (Myambutol) can cause optic neuritis. What visual changes might this include? *(Select all that apply.)*
    ____ A. Double vision
    ____ B. Red-green color blindness
    ____ C. Reduced visual fields
    ____ D. Reduced color vision
    ____ E. Blurred vision
    ____ F. Reduced central vision

____ 2. Before administering rifampin (RIF) you should assess for an allergy to which substance?
    A. Sulfonamides
    B. Aspirin
    C. Sulfites
    D. Penicillin

____ 3. Which statement demonstrates that a patient understands the precautions necessary when taking rifampin (RIF) while on oral contraceptives?
    A. "As long as I don't miss any doses, I will be protected."
    B. "My partner will use condoms until I have finished with the drug."
    C. "I will take two oral contraceptive pills a day instead of just one."
    D. "I will use a second method until one month after I finish taking the rifampin."

____ 4. First-line antitubercular drugs are indicated for which patient?
   A. Pregnant female, to prevent TB infection
   B. Older male taking lipid-lowering medication
   C. Pregnant female with active TB
   D. Nursing mother

5. A patient with coccidioidomycosis has the antifungal drug amphotericin B (Fungizone) prescribed. Which are serious adverse effects of this medication? *(Select all that apply.)*
   ____ A. Reduced kidney function
   ____ B. Hypercalcemia
   ____ C. Bowel obstruction
   ____ D. Widespread skin flushing
   ____ E. Fever and chills

____ 6. Before administering an azole antifungal agent, what should the nurse plan to do?
   A. Administer the medication with grapefruit juice.
   B. Administer the medication with a histamine blocker.
   C. Give the medication at a different time as a proton pump inhibitor.
   D. Premedicate the patient with acetaminophen or ibuprofen.

____ 7. Which patient teaching point is important to include for a patient taking ketoconazole (Nizoral)?
   A. Apply suntan lotion before using tanning beds.
   B. Wear protective clothing when in the sun.
   C. Restrict fluids to decrease the likelihood of kidney impairment.
   D. Apply antiembolism stockings to prevent deep vein thrombosis.

____ 8. A child with tinea capitis has been prescribed terbinafine (Lamisil). The child should have this medication administered in which manner?
   A. To the scalp
   B. To the feet
   C. In the groin area
   D. Orally

____ 9. Which diet recommendation is most crucial to provide for a patient who is taking isoniazid, to prevent peripheral neuropathy?
   A. Decrease saturated fats and cholesterol.
   B. Increase the intake of B vitamins.
   C. Eat foods that are higher in iron and calcium.
   D. Decrease foods that contain uric acids.

____ 10. A patient who is receiving amphotericin B is also receiving intravenous corticosteroids to reduce which possible adverse effect?
   A. Skin itching
   B. Fever and chills
   C. Decreased kidney function
   D. Blood vessel dilation

Drugs Affecting the Immune System

LEARNING ACTIVITIES

Matching: Terminology Review

Match each definition with the corresponding term. (Use each term only once, not all terms will be used.)

____ 1. Type of antibody-mediated immunity a person has if antibodies made by another person against an antigen are injected into the body

____ 2. Vaccine composed of science-made substances that are very similar to the parts of a virus or bacterium that causes disease

____ 3. A vaccine composed of organisms that could cause diseases but have been killed or inactivated by heat, radiation, or chemicals

____ 4. Vaccine that contains live organisms that have been modified so they are no longer capable of causing disease

____ 5. The type of antibody-mediated immunity that is started when a person is invaded by a foreign organism without assistance, and B cells learn to make antibodies against the invaders

____ 6. Type of antibody-mediated immunity started when an antigen is deliberately placed into the body to force B cells to make a specific antibody against it

____ 7. A vaccine that contains either a modified toxin that an organism produces or an actual part of the organism

____ 8. Type of antibody-mediated immunity acquired as a result of antibodies transferred to a fetus or infant from the mother through the placenta and through breast milk

A. Artificially acquired active immunity
B. Naturally acquired active immunity
C. Toxoid
D. Artificially acquired passive immunity
E. Naturally acquired passive immunity
F. True immunity
G. Inactivated vaccine
H. Attenuated vaccine
I. Biosynthetic vaccine

Fill in the Blank

9. A human will not develop distemper because of _____ immunity.

10. Any cell, product, or protein with a code different than your own that enters your body and is recognized by the immune system as foreign is a(n) _____ to you.

11. _____ and _____ are examples of attenu-
    ated vaccines.

12. A person who travels to an area of the world where contagious dis-
    eases are more common should receive specific vaccinations against
    _____, _____, _____, and
    _____.

13. A patient believes she has been exposed to chickenpox, but does not
    remember if she had the disease as a child. The patient can have a(n)
    _____ _____ blood level drawn to deter-
    mine if she is protected against the disease.

14. Disease-modifying antirheumatic drugs (DMARDs) reduce disease pro-
    gression and tissue destruction by inhibiting _____
    _____ _____.

15. _____ _____ act by purposely destroying
    cells.

16. Mycophenolate reversibly inhibits a(n) _____ needed for
    lymphocyte reproduction and prevents T-cells already present from being ac-
    tive.

17. Polyclonal antibodies are produced by other animals, such as
    _____ and _____.

18. All selective immunosuppressants can cause the patient to be at an increased
    risk for _____.

19. The pharmacy employee who is mixing antiproliferative drugs is using
    personal protective equipment because the drug can be absorbed through
    _____ and _____ _____.

MEDICATION SAFETY PRACTICE

1. A pregnant woman should NOT receive which vaccines?

2. A child who has undergone a kidney transplant is to receive azathioprine
   (Imuran) 2 mg/kg orally every day. The child weighs 78 pounds. How much
   of the drug should the child receive?

3. A drug in the category of antiproliferatives can cause failure of which major
   organ system?

4. Which equipment should be nearby when monoclonal or polyclonal antibodies are being administered? Why?

5. A patient has undergone a liver transplant. What four areas of instruction should be provided to maintain the effectiveness of the immunosuppressant drugs?

6. Which instructions are most crucial to provide for a patient taking sirolimus or cyclosporine?

PRACTICE QUIZ

___ 1. A patient taking oral sirolimus has been provided instructions on how to take the medication. Which patient statement indicates the need for further instruction?
A. "I can disguise the flavor of this medication by mixing it with grapefruit juice."
B. "I can take this medication with a meal if needed to prevent stomach upset."
C. "If I take this medication at 8 AM, I can take the cyclosporine at 1 PM."
D. "I should follow the mixing instructions on the label provided by the pharmacist."

___ 2. A woman who had an organ transplant is taking an antiproliferative agent, and is now considering having a child. Which patient instruction is most important to provide?
A. "You are not as likely to reject the new organ while you are pregnant."
B. "You should use two reliable methods of contraception while on this drug."
C. "If you do get pregnant, consider breastfeeding to provide immunity to the baby."
D. "If you stop taking the medications, you may begin your pregnancy right away."

___ 3. Which diseases are most likely to be treated with DMARDs? *(Select all that apply.)*
___ A. Crohn's disease
___ B. Peptic ulcers
___ C. Pseudomembranous colitis
___ D. Psoriatic arthritis
___ E. Ankylosing spondylitis

___ 4. Which immunizations should be provided to an older adult? *(Select all that apply.)*
___ A. Measles
___ B. Pneumonia
___ C. Shingles
___ D. Seasonal influenza
___ E. Polio

___ 5. A parent brings a 2-week-old infant to the pediatrician and says, "I've been worried about the pertussis outbreak. When is the earliest my baby should get the pertussis vaccine?" Which should be the nurse's answer?
A. "It can be given today."
B. "When the baby is 1 year old."
C. "When the baby is 6 months old."
D. "When the baby is 2 months old."

___ 6. Which is an example of a toxoid vaccine?
A. Rubella
B. Measles
C. Tetanus
D. Chickenpox

____ 7. Breastfeeding an infant is encouraged because it provides the infant with which type of immunity?
   A. Naturally acquired active immunity
   B. Naturally acquired passive immunity
   C. Artificially acquired active immunity
   D. Artificially acquired passive immunity

____ 8. At age 11, a patient contracted measles when his brothers and sisters also had the disease. This patient will be immune for a long time due to which type of immunity?
   A. Naturally acquired active immunity
   B. Naturally acquired passive immunity
   C. Artificially acquired active immunity
   D. Artificially acquired passive immunity

____ 9. In a clinic that provides immunizations, you see a vial of last year's flu vaccine that is not expired. Even though the vial has not expired, you cannot administer it this year for which reason?
   A. The expiration dating system is not accurate and is not likely to be reliable.
   B. A new vaccine is developed annually for viruses predicted to be prevalent this year.
   C. Last year's vaccine would likely cause a very severe drug allergy or anaphylaxis.
   D. Third-party insurers will not cover vaccines that should have been given last year.

____ 10. A patient is taking a calcineurin inhibitor drug. This patient will need to be monitored for liver toxicity by observing for which sign?
   A. Redness of the conjunctival sac
   B. Cloudiness over the pupils of the eye
   C. Yellowing of the sclera of the eye
   D. Purulent drainage mixed with tears

____ 11. A patient taking polyclonal antibodies should be questioned about allergies to which animal prior to taking the medication?
   A. Birds
   B. Cats
   C. Horses
   D. Dogs

Anticancer Drugs

LEARNING ACTIVITIES

Matching: Terminology Review

Match the definitions on the right with their correct terms on the left. (Answers will be used only once.)

____ 1. Apoptosis

____ 2. Benign

____ 3. Carcinogen

____ 4. Cyclins

____ 5. Emetogenic

____ 6. Extravasation

____ 7. Suppressor gene product

____ 8. Cancer arising from glandular tissue

____ 9. Metastasis

____ 10. Mitosis

____ 11. Mucositis

____ 12. Cytotoxic

____ 13. Neutropenia

____ 14. Primary tumor

____ 15. Thrombocytopenia

____ 16. Vesicant

A. Reduced number of platelets
B. Spread of cancer cells to other body areas
C. Normal cells dividing
D. Severe white blood cell suppression
E. Carcinoma
F. Tumor type that is usually harmless
G. Inflammation and ulcers in mucous membranes
H. Substance or event that can cause cancer development
I. Chemicals or drugs that damage tissue on direct contact
J. Limits cell division
K. Programmed cell death
L. Proteins promoting cells to divide
M. Substance that induces vomiting
N. Leakage of irritating drug into surrounding tissues
O. Cell-damaging and cell-killing effects
P. Original site where normal cells become cancer

Matching

Match the mechanism of action on the right with its correct chemotherapy drug category on the left. (Answers will be used only once.)

____ 17. Antimetabolites

____ 18. Antitumor antibiotics

____ 19. Antimitotics

____ 20. Alkylating agents

____ 21. Topoisomerase inhibitors

A. Interfere with tubule formation
B. Cause DNA breakage and cell death
C. Fool cancer cells into using the wrong substance in cellular reactions
D. Bind DNA strands by cross-linking
E. Interrupt synthesis of DNA or RNA

Fill in the Blank

22. A patient receiving interleukins may have a generalized, severe inflammatory reaction, resulting in _____ forming in most tissues.

23. Thalidomide is contraindicated during _____.

24. Colony-stimulating factors may stimulate the growth of _____ cells.

25. Cell division is rapid and continuous in _____ cells.

26. Cancer cells tend to grow in a way that is _____ and _____.

Multiple Choice

27. Which drugs might be administered before chemotherapy as premedications? *(Select all that apply.)*
    _____ A. prochlorperazine (Compazine)
    _____ B. dexamethasone (Decadron)
    _____ C. lorazepam (Ativan)
    _____ D. nicotinic acid (Niacin)
    _____ E. cephalexin (Keflex)
    _____ F. metformin (Glucophage)

Matching: Physiology and Pathophysiology of Cancer

Match the features associated with normal cells, benign tumors, and cancer cells. (Each term may be used more than once.)

_____ 28. Grow by expansion

_____ 29. Have an anaplastic appearance

_____ 30. Respond to signals for apoptosis

_____ 31. Serve no useful purpose

_____ 32. Represent normal tissue growing in the wrong place

_____ 33. Divide only when body conditions and nutrition are just right

_____ 34. Have orderly growth that is not needed for normal function

_____ 35. Reenter the cell cycle almost as fast as they complete it

_____ 36. Have specific, differentiated functions needed for whole-body function

_____ 37. Grow by invasion

_____ 38. Are very loosely adherent

_____ 39. Spend most of their lives in the state of G_0

A. Benign tumors
B. Cancer cells
C. Normal cells

Matching: Chemotherapy Drug Categories

Indicate whether the following chemotherapy drugs are classified as alkylating agents, topoisomerase inhibitors, or miscellaneous chemotherapy drugs (other agents). (Each term may be used more than once.)

_____ 40. oxaliplatin (Eloxatin)

_____ 41. procarbazine (Matulane)

_____ 42. busulfan (Myleran)

_____ 43. temozolomide (Temodar)

_____ 44. asparaginase (Elspar)

_____ 45. topotecan (Hycamtin)

_____ 46. cisplatin (Platinol)

_____ 47. melphalan (Alkeran)

_____ 48. irinotecan (Camptosar)

_____ 49. hydroxyurea (Hydrea)

_____ 50. pegaspargase (Oncaspar)

_____ 51. cyclophosphamide (Cytoxan)

A. Alkylating agent
B. Miscellaneous chemotherapy drug
C. Topoisomerase inhibitor

MEDICATION SAFETY PRACTICE

1. Due to the risk of absorption of chemotherapy drugs, what precautions must be taken in preparation and administration? *(Select all that apply.)*
   _____ A. Eye protection
   _____ B. Mask
   _____ C. Foot covering
   _____ D. Hair covering
   _____ E. Double gloves
   _____ F. Laminar flow hood
   _____ G. Gown
   _____ H. Prophylactic interferon injections

_____ 2. In the event of an adverse or anaphylactic reaction during the administration of chemotherapy drugs, what is the priority action?
   A. Notify the primary care provider.
   B. Administer diphenhydramine (Benadryl).
   C. Prevent any more drug from entering the patient.
   D. Slow the infusion to a "keep open" rate.
   E. Discontinue the IV and apply warm packs.

3. What teaching interventions are required for a patient who has thrombocytopenia? *(Select all that apply.)*
   _____ A. Drink at least 2 liters of fluid daily.
   _____ B. Avoid dairy products.
   _____ C. Use a soft-bristled toothbrush.
   _____ D. Avoid straining with bowel movements.
   _____ E. Use enemas or suppositories to prevent constipation.
   _____ F. Maintain a daily aspirin regimen.
   _____ G. Consult the oncologist before scheduling any dental work.

PRACTICE QUIZ

_____ 1. Which regimen of antiemetics is most likely to control chemotherapy-induced nausea and vomiting?
  A. Start with prochlorperazine (Compazine) and move to more potent drugs such as ondansetron (Zofran) or granisetron (Kytril) as needed.
  B. Administer medications on a PRN basis, not exceeding the maximum recommended dosage.
  C. Premedicate before chemotherapy administration and continue the medication on a scheduled basis.
  D. Alternate oral and parenteral routes of administration to maximize drug absorption.

_____ 2. A patient who is receiving chemotherapy is fatigued and has an oxygen saturation of 86%. The patient's red blood cell count is 1.8 million/mm³. After starting supplemental oxygen, what treatment is the prescriber most likely to order?
  A. Plasmapheresis
  B. Bone marrow transplant
  C. Platelet cell transfusion
  D. Biologic response modifier

3. Which are known carcinogens? (_Select all that apply._)
  _____ A. Tobacco
  _____ B. Radiation
  _____ C. Measles virus
  _____ D. Human papilloma virus
  _____ E. Varicella virus

_____ 4. Which is a life-threatening and common reason a patient's chemotherapy session would be postponed or rescheduled?
  A. Thrombocytopenia
  B. Alopecia
  C. Mucositis
  D. Cognitive function changes

_____ 5. A patient who has had treatment for breast cancer should be monitored for the spread of cancer to which area?
  A. Gastrointestinal tract
  B. Lungs
  C. Pancreas
  D. Pelvis

_____ 6. A patient with cancer wants to postpone several appointments for chemotherapy. Postponement is discouraged because the basis for scheduling chemotherapy doses is dependent on which factor?
  A. Available transportation for the patient
  B. Doctor's schedule
  C. Availability of medication from the manufacturer
  D. Maximization of cancer cells killed

_____ 7. In an oncology clinic, several patients' pathology reports are being reviewed by the health care team. Which description is most likely to apply to cancer cells?
  A. No differentiated function
  B. Tight adherence
  C. Nonmigration
  D. Well-regulated growth

_____ 8. A patient is receiving chemotherapy through a peripheral IV site. Which action will most likely prevent extravasation?
  A. Apply cool compresses over the IV site during infusion.
  B. Assess the IV infusion site at least every 30 minutes.
  C. Discontinue the infusion if a brisk blood return is present.
  D. Ensure that only an advanced-practice registered nurse gives the medication.

_____ 9. A patient who has undergone chemotherapy has received instruction about how to avoid infections if neutropenia develops. Which patient statement indicates a need for further teaching?
  A. "I will ask someone else in my household to clean the cat litterbox."
  B. "I should not dig in my garden or work with house plants."
  C. "I will need to avoid eating raw fresh fruits and vegetables."
  D. "I will need a platelet transfusion if my counts remain low."

_____ 10. Which is essential to include when teaching patients about thrombocytopenia?
   A. Playing football is acceptable if the patient wears a helmet and padding.
   B. A white blood cell transfusion may be necessary if the counts remain low.
   C. Do not have dental work performed without consulting your oncologist.
   D. Use enemas or rectal suppositories to relieve occasional constipation.

_____ 11. A woman is undergoing treatment for cancer and is receiving thalidomide. She would like to start a pregnancy. What advice is most appropriate?
   A. "You have more important things to think about than pregnancy."
   B. "You should use at least two forms of contraception to avoid pregnancy."
   C. "Pregnancy would likely improve your mood and outlook toward cancer."
   D. "Thalidomide is safer during the first trimester, while the embryo is small."

_____ 12. Hormone manipulation therapy is most frequently prescribed for patients who have which type of cancer?
   A. Prostate
   B. Liver
   C. Lung
   D. Bone

_____ 13. A patient with melanoma will be receiving interferon therapy. What is the expected benefit from this drug?
   A. It helps cancer cells appear abnormal.
   B. It increases the expression of oncogenes.
   C. It increases cell division within tumors.
   D. It stimulates growth of natural killer cells.

_____ 14. Targeted therapies combine which aspects of treatment?
   A. Gene therapy and immunotherapy
   B. Cell growth inhibition and carcinogen suppression
   C. Antimetabolites and antimitotic effects
   D. Alkylating activity and antitumor antibody production

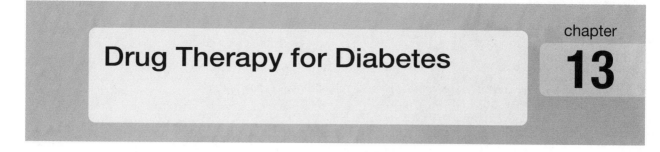

Drug Therapy for Diabetes

chapter
13

LEARNING ACTIVITIES

Crossword Puzzle: Terminology Review

Complete the puzzle by identifying the correct terms described in the clues below.

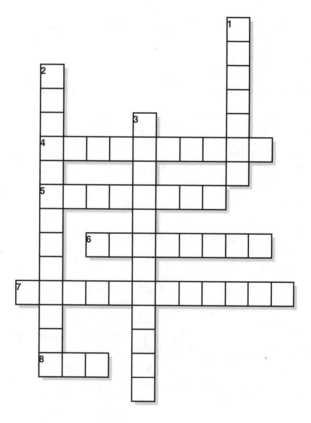

Across
4. Normal range of fasting blood glucose
5. Hormone secreted by pancreas alpha cells
6. Type of diabetes related to reduced insulin effectiveness
7. Excessive byproduct of fat metabolism
8. Body's main chemical energy substance

Down
1. Hormone secreted by pancreas beta cells
2. Higher-than-normal blood glucose level
3. Lower-than-normal blood glucose level

Fill in the Blank

Fill in the blank with the correct term regarding possible complications of poorly controlled diabetes.

1. _____ blood cholesterol levels

2. _____ risk for heart attack

3. _____ wound healing

4. Loss of _____ sensation

5. _____ failure

6. Erectile _____

Fill in the blank with the correct information about the types and durations of insulin

7. Peak time of insulin aspart (NovoLog) _____

8. Duration of action of regular insulin (Humulin) _____

9. Onset of isophane insulin NPH (Novolin N) _____

10. Duration of action of insulin glargine (Lantus) _____

Matching

Match each type of oral antidiabetic drug on the right with its correct drug name on the left. (Drug types will be used more than once.)

_____ 11. pioglitazone (Actos)

_____ 12. glipizide (Glucotrol)

_____ 13. repaglinide (Prandin)

_____ 14. glyburide (DiaBeta, Micronase)

_____ 15. acarbose (Precose)

_____ 16. glimepiride (Amaryl)

_____ 17. nateglinide (Starlix)

_____ 18. glyburide, micronized (Glynase)

_____ 19. metformin (Glucophage)

_____ 20. miglitol (Glyset)

_____ 21. rosiglitazone (Avandia)

_____ 22. exenatide (Byetta)

_____ 23. pramlintide (Symlin)

_____ 24. liraglutide (Victoza)

A. Sulfonylurea
B. Meglitinide
C. Biguanide
D. Alpha-glucosidase inhibitor
E. Thiazolidinedione
F. Incretin mimetic
G. Amylin analogs

Matching: Pathophysiology of Diabetes

Indicate which symptoms, complications, and management strategies are associated with type 1 diabetes, type 2 diabetes, or both type 1 and type 2 diabetes. (Answers will be used more than once.)

____ 25. Hyperglycemia is present.

____ 26. Onset of symptoms is sudden.

____ 27. Symptoms most commonly begin in adults over age 40.

____ 28. Always requires insulin for treatment.

____ 29. The risks for heart disease and kidney disease are increased.

____ 30. More likely to occur in people who are overweight.

____ 31. Ketoacidosis is a serious complication.

____ 32. The most common type of diabetes mellitus.

____ 33. The patient has an increased risk for infection.

____ 34. A major symptom before treatment is started is increased thirst.

____ 35. The patient still makes some of his or her own insulin.

____ 36. Hypertension is common.

A. Type 1 diabetes
B. Type 2 diabetes
C. Type 1 and type 2 diabetes

MEDICATION SAFETY PRACTICE

1. The patient will be instructed to rotate injection sites for insulin to minimize the risk of developing _____ _____.

2. True or False: After inserting the needle for an insulin injection, aspiration should be done before depressing the plunger.

3. True or False: Before withdrawing insulin from the bottle or using a prefilled device, the container should be shaken vigorously to make sure the suspension is evenly distributed.

4. True or False: Prefilled pens and cartridges of insulin detemir (Levemir) should be stored at room temperature.

5. List three challenges to maintaining good control over blood glucose levels in pediatric patients.

    a. _____

    b. _____

    c. _____

6. What actions are important to take *after* giving a patient a noninsulin antidiabetic drug?

   a. _____

   b. _____

   c. _____

PRACTICE QUIZ

____ 1. What effect are the last two trimesters of pregnancy likely to have on the insulin needs of a patient with diabetes?
A. Increase during morning hours
B. Decrease at bedtime
C. Plateau at lunchtime
D. Overall increase

____ 2. Which conditions can result from poorly controlled diabetes? *(Select all that apply.)*
____ A. Increased risk for infection
____ B. Increased sensitivity to touch
____ C. Elevated cholesterol levels
____ D. Kidney failure
____ E. Orthostatic hypotension

____ 3. A patient with diabetes who takes glucophage (Metformin) has postoperative orders to "resume all preoperative medications." What is the priority action to take?
A. Follow the orders and resume all preoperative medications.
B. Hold all preoperative medications until verified with the pharmacy.
C. Contact the prescriber to obtain an order to hold the glucophage for 48 hours.
D. Resume only oral preoperative medications.
E. Hold oral preoperative medications until the patient has a bowel movement.

____ 4. A 68-year-old patient who is taking pioglitazone (Actos) will have which laboratory test done for follow-up?
A. Pulmonary function test (PFT)
B. Alanine transaminase (ALT)
C. Thyroid-stimulating hormone (TSH)
D. Complete blood count (CBC)

____ 5. A patient has been prescribed exenatide (Byetta). Which patient statement indicates a correct understanding of the use of this drug?
A. "I should keep this medication in the refrigerator, not the freezer."
B. "Even if I miss breakfast, I should still take my exenatide."
C. "This medication can cause weight gain, so I'll need to eat less."
D. "This medication can cause me to feel hungrier between meals."

____ 6. At 10 AM, a patient who was given an injection of Humulin R at 7:30 AM is anxious, has cool clammy skin, and noticeable hand tremors. What is the most likely explanation for these symptoms?
A. The insulin is nearing the end of its duration of action.
B. The insulin is having its peak effect, causing hypoglycemia.
C. The patient likely ingested an excessive amount of carbohydrates.
D. The patient has received an insufficient amount of insulin.

____ 7. Which is the best action to ensure proper dosing before administering 50 units of Humulin N?
A. Use a 5-mL syringe and administer 0.5 mL.
B. Administer 50 units of insulin glargine.
C. Ensure the vial contents are completely clear.
D. Use a 50-unit or a 100-unit syringe.

Drug Therapy for Thyroid and Adrenal Gland Problems

chapter
14

LEARNING ACTIVITIES

Crossword Puzzle: Terminology Review

Complete the puzzle by identifying the correct words described in the clues below.

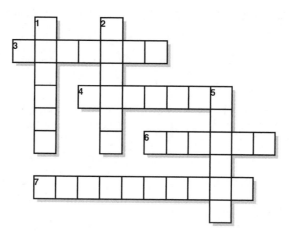

Across
3. An endocrine glands secretes a(n) _____.
4. The adrenal glands are located on top of the _____.
6. The target tissue of estrogen is the _____.
7. Thyroid hormones increase the rate of _____.

Down
1. The thick outermost layer of the adrenal gland is known as the _____.
2. Saltwater fish is a common dietary source of _____.
5. Cortisol (glucocorticoid) regulates the body's response to _____.

Fill in the Blank

1. Aminoglutethimide (Cytadren) works by directly inhibiting the _____ gland production of _____.

2. A medication to suppress adrenal hormone production is effective if the blood levels of _____ and _____ are reduced.

3. _____ is a hormone secreted by the adrenal cortex that regulates sodium and water balance.

4. _____ _____ _____ is a drug that mimics the effect of thyroid hormones to help regulate metabolism.

5. _____ are drugs similar to natural cortisol, a hormone secreted by the adrenal cortex that is essential for life.

6. A tissue or organ that is affected or controlled by the hormone is a(n) _____ _____.

7. The two thyroid hormones produced by the thyroid are _____ and _____.

8. _____ _____ and _____ _____ are common dietary sources of iodine.

9. _____ is the energy use of each cell, and the amount of work performed in the body.

10. Thyroid gland cells can divide, making the thyroid gland larger, causing a swelling in the neck called a(n) _____.

11. _____ is a severe type of hypothyroidism, which requires immediate medical attention.

12. Thyrotoxicosis is another term for _____ thyroid hormones.

Matching: Thyroid Disorders

Match the signs and symptoms with the correct thyroid disorder. (Answers will be used more than once.)

_____ 13. Sleeping excessively

_____ 14. Facial edema

_____ 15. Feeling warm most of the time

_____ 16. Rapid heart rate

_____ 17. Weight gain

_____ 18. Slowed speech

_____ 19. Diarrhea

_____ 20. Slow respiratory rate

A. Hypothyroidism
B. Hyperthyroidism

Matching: Thyroid Hormone Replacement Drugs

Indicate whether the following precautions should or should not be taught to patients who are taking thyroid hormone replacement drugs. (Answers will be used more than once.)

_____ 21. Do not take these drugs during pregnancy.

_____ 22. You can skip these drugs for up to a week if you are on vacation or do not feel well.

_____ 23. Do not take a higher dose of the drug than what has been prescribed for you.

_____ 24. Do not breastfeed an infant while taking these drugs.

_____ 25. Go to the emergency department immediately if you have chest pain.

_____ 26. If constipation occurs, stop the drug immediately.

_____ 27. Take these drugs 3 hours before or 4 hours after taking a fiber supplement.

_____ 28. These drugs enhance the activity of warfarin and increase the risk for excessive bleeding.

_____ 29. These drugs decrease the activity of warfarin and increase the risk for blood clot formation.

_____ 30. These drugs reduce the effectiveness of oral contraceptives.

A. Should teach
B. Should not teach

MEDICATION SAFETY PRACTICE

1. A patient is being educated about the interaction between thyroid hormone replacement drugs and warfarin (Coumadin) because of the increased risk of

   _____.

2. Thyroid hormone replacement drugs should never be substituted for one another due to their variation in strengths, as well as the patient's

   _____.

3. A female patient who is of childbearing age and taking mifepristone is cautioned to use two forms of reliable contraception, because the drug can cause

   _____ _____.

4. A child who weighs 22 pounds is prescribed levothyroxine (Levothroid) 10 mcg/kg daily. How many mcg will the child receive each day? _____ mcg

5. A patient who is taking a thyroid hormone should be advised to take the drug at what time in regard to food or fiber supplement?

PRACTICE QUIZ

_____ 1. Which statement by a patient who is taking thyroid replacement medication demonstrates a correct understanding of the therapy?
  A. "As soon as my levels get back to normal, I can quit taking these pills."
  B. "These pills will only serve to make me gain weight."
  C. "I hope to feel better in general, and be more energetic during the day."
  D. "I'll take this in the evening when I take my fiber supplement; that way I won't forget."

2. What cardiac events may result from increased activity brought about by thyroid hormone replacement? *(Select all that apply.)*
  _____ A. Tamponade
  _____ B. Infarction
  _____ C. Heart block
  _____ D. Angina
  _____ E. Aortic stenosis
  _____ F. Heart failure

_____ 3. A patient who has Graves' disease has an endocrine disorder characterized by what action?
  A. The thyroid gland does not produce enough hormone.
  B. The body makes antibodies to thyroid-stimulating hormone, which bind to receptors.
  C. Antigens produced in the blood block hormone function.
  D. Slowed body metabolism causes decreased production of thyroid hormone.

_____ 4. Which statement best describes the mechanism of action of thyroid-suppressing drugs?
  A. Cells in the thyroid gland are killed by toxins and rendered unable to produce hormone.
  B. Thiamine is destroyed and cannot connect with iodine to make hormone.
  C. Hormones already formed and stored in the gland are depleted.
  D. The drug combines with the enzyme responsible for connecting iodide with tyrosine.

_____ 5. Before administering thyroid replacement hormones, which action is crucial?
  A. Administering the medication on the same schedule as at home
  B. Encouraging the patient to ask the pharmacist for a less-expensive brand
  C. Administering the medication with food to decrease stomach upset
  D. Dividing the prescribed medication into several doses throughout the day

_____ 6. An infant has been diagnosed with congenital absence of the thyroid gland. What should be emphasized during parent counseling?
  A. Most thyroid medications are prepared from nonallergenic animals.
  B. This medication is prescribed to promote mental and physical development.
  C. This medication will need to be taken only through adolescence.
  D. This medication eliminates the need for future monitoring of thyroid levels.

_____ 7. A patient asks, "How will I know when the thyroid replacement medication is working?" Which is the best response?
  A. "When your heart rate and blood pressure begin to decrease."
  B. "You probably will feel dramatically different within a week."
  C. "You will likely experience less constipation than previously."
  D. "You may begin to feel drowsier than you normally feel."

_____ 8. A patient with a history of a seizure disorder has had thyroid hormone recently prescribed. What precautions should be in place for this person?
  A. The patient should stop taking the thyroid hormone replacement.
  B. The patient will likely not experience any more seizures.
  C. The patient should take half of the prescribed antiseizure medications.
  D. The patient should be monitored for a higher risk of seizures.

_____ 9. The parent of a child who has had hypothyroidism since birth remarks, "He's gone through three shoe sizes in six months; he must be on a growth spurt!" What is an important aspect of care with thyroid replacement hormone treatment during rapid growth stages?

A. The child will need an increase in the amount of replacement hormone.

B. The child will be able to stop taking the thyroid replacement hormone.

C. Growth spurts are common during childhood; no changes are needed.

D. Further testing will likely now reveal the thyroid tissue has regrown.

10. A patient with hyperthyroidism is to be monitored for symptoms of a thyroid crisis. Which symptoms are associated with this disorder? _(Select all that apply.)_

_____ A. Hypothermia

_____ B. Slow pulse

_____ C. Hypertension

_____ D. Fever

_____ E. Lethargy

_____ 11. A patient who is pregnant has been diagnosed with hyperthyroidism. What will likely be included in the patient's plan of care?

A. The patient will be able to take additional doses of thyroid replacement hormone.

B. Thyroid-suppressing medications are not generally prescribed during pregnancy.

C. The patient will be able to take thyroid-suppressing drugs once she starts breastfeeding.

D. The pregnant patient will be at a higher risk of infection, making surgical treatment unsafe.

_____ 12. Which is an assessment finding associated with adrenal gland hypofunction?

A. Puffy, swollen facial features

B. "Buffalo hump" noted on the back

C. Overdeveloped muscles

D. Darkening of the skin

_____ 13. Fludrocortisone (Florinef) is expected to cause which change?

A. Lower the sodium level

B. Reduce the potassium level

C. Lower the blood pressure

D. Lower the blood sugar

_____ 14. A patient taking an adrenal hormone-suppressing drug, mitotane (Lysodren) should have which change when the medication becomes effective?

A. Normal growth pattern established

B. Normal hair growth in place

C. Reduced blood level of aldosterone

D. Improved menstrual regularity

_____ 15. An older adult is taking thyroid suppressing medication. Which is an important consideration for this patient?

A. Instruct the patient that blood clots are more likely to form

B. Recognize there is an increased risk for infection

C. The effects of warfarin are decreased

D. Adverse effects are less likely to be severe

Drug Therapy Affecting Urine Output

LEARNING ACTIVITIES

Matching

Match the correct category of drug on the right with the name of the drug on the left. (Answers will be used more than once.)

____ 1. oxybutynin (Detrol)

____ 2. solifenacin (Vesicare)

____ 3. hydrochlorothiazide (Microzide)

____ 4. torsemide (Demadex)

____ 5. metolazone (Zaroxolyn)

____ 6. spironolactone (Aldactone)

____ 7. furosemide (Lasix)

____ 8. trospium chloride (Sanctura XR)

____ 9. darifenacin (Enablex)

____ 10. bumetanide (Bumex)

____ 11. ethacrynic acid (Edecrin)

A. Diuretic
B. Urinary antispasmodic

Fill in the Blank

Fill in the blanks for each question with the correct answers.

12. A natriuretic diuretic is one that causes excretion of _____ and _____ in the urine.

13. The part of the kidney where filtration takes place is the _____.

14. The detrusor muscle squeezes urine from the _____ into the _____.

15. Diuretics should be taken in the morning to decrease the incidence of _____.

16. The patient taking potassium-sparing diuretics should be aware of these signs of an increased potassium level: _____, _____, _____, and _____.

MEDICATION SAFETY PRACTICE

_____ 1.   What is the correct daily oral dose (in milligrams) of furosemide (Lasix)
           for a child who weighs 20 pounds?
           A. 10.18
           B. 18.2
           C. 20
           D. 40

_____ 2.   Which beverage should a patient taking bumetanide (Bumex) avoid?
           A. Grapefruit juice
           B. Milk
           C. Wine
           D. Green tea

_____ 3.   A patient taking a loop diuretic should report which symptom as an
           early indication of ototoxicity?
           A. Decreased urine output
           B. "Ringing" in the ears
           C. "Popping" sounds in the ears
           D. Hearing voices no one else can hear

_____ 4.   Which fall prevention intervention should be in place for a patient tak-
           ing a potassium-sparing diuretic?
           A. Assist the patient to move slowly from a sitting to a standing posi-
               tion.
           B. Leave oranges, bananas, and grapefruit close within the patient's
               reach.
           C. Discuss the possibility of vest restraint devices with the health care
               provider.
           D. Suggest the patient remain in bed while taking this medication.

_____ 5.   A patient is taking oxybutynin gel packets to treat overactive bladder.
           She should be advised to avoid which activity?
           A. Walking too far away from a bathroom
           B. Taking the medication at night
           C. Exercising in hot, humid weather
           D. Using the topical gel on the upper arms

PRACTICE QUIZ

_____ 1.   A patient taking a potassium-sparing di-
           uretic should be monitored for which side
           effect?
           A. Gynecomastia
           B. Alopecia
           C. Hypertension
           D. Hyperglycemia

_____ 2.   A patient is being evaluated for treatment
           with hydrochlorothiazide (Microzide).
           Which laboratory value warrants notifica-
           tion to the prescriber?
           A. Urine specific gravity of less than
               1.0028
           B. Serum white blood cell (WBC) count
               greater than 4000/mm^3
           C. Potassium below 3 mEq/L
           D. Serum creatinine of 1 mg/dL

____ 3. Which question is relevant in evaluating a patient who is taking bumetanide (Bumex) in combination with gentamicin (Garamycin)?
   A. "What is the date today?"
   B. "How many fingers do you see?"
   C. "Can you hear this whisper?"
   D. "Can you touch your index finger to your nose?"

4. Which statements best demonstrate a patient's understanding of treatment with tolterodine (Detrol)? *(Select all that apply.)*
   ____ A. "I need to decrease my fluid intake while I am on this medication."
   ____ B. "My husband is going to drive until I see how this drug will affect me."
   ____ C. "I will change the patch every day."
   ____ D. "I will call the doctor if I get a rash where the patch has been."
   ____ E. "This drug will help stop the sudden need to go that I've been having."

5. A patient is taking 20 mg of metolazone (Zaroxolyn) by mouth daily to reduce edema. Before discharge, the patient will be taught which instructions? *(Select all that apply.)*
   ____ A. Slowly change positions from lying to sitting and sitting to standing.
   ____ B. Limit fluid intake to 1 liter per day.
   ____ C. Increased saliva production can be managed by reducing water intake.
   ____ D. Wear sunscreen and appropriate clothing to avoid sunburn.
   ____ E. Use caution in tasks that require mental activity and muscle strength.

____ 6. What instruction should be given to a patient who is taking hydrochlorothiazide (Microzide) and potassium when nausea develops?
   A. "Hold the potassium until the nausea is over."
   B. "Take the potassium even though you are nauseated to avoid heart problems."
   C. "Decrease the amount of potassium to every other day until you feel better."
   D. "Decrease the amount of diuretic and the amount of potassium by one-half for one day."

7. An older adult is taking furosemide (Lasix). Which special precautions are necessary for this patient? *(Select all that apply.)*
   ____ A. Report new onset of muscle weakness to the prescriber.
   ____ B. Elevated potassium levels may result from this medication.
   ____ C. Instruct the patient to sit on the side of the bed before standing up.
   ____ D. Hearing loss and tinnitus can be associated with the use of furosemide.
   ____ E. Older adults are less sensitive to the effects of furosemide.

____ 8. A pregnant woman should be given which advice regarding thiazide diuretics?
   A. The medication can cause increased fetal potassium levels.
   B. The medication can be taken to lower blood pressure during pregnancy.
   C. It is best to wait until breastfeeding to resume taking this medication.
   D. This medication is associated with jaundice in the newborn.

____ 9. A patient who has diabetes should be provided which instruction while taking furosemide (Lasix)?
   A. Eat an additional 300-500 calories a day to avoid blood sugar decreases.
   B. Monitor your blood sugar more closely for an increase.
   C. You may be more sensitive to rapid drops in your blood sugar level.
   D. Your health care provider will likely suggest a decrease in your insulin dose.

____ 10. Which is important to include in patient teaching for an older adult who is taking a loop diuretic?
   A. Avoid fruits such as bananas, oranges, and grapefruit in your diet.
   B. Increase the amount of foods containing fiber to avoid constipation.
   C. You may be at higher risk of falling while taking this medication.
   D. Hearing loss is a common occurrence during aging and is not concerning.

____ 11. A female patient who is taking spironolactone (Aldactone) should be advised of which common side effect?
   A. Development of hirsutism
   B. Shrinkage of breast tissue
   C. Premenstrual syndrome
   D. Decreased voice loudness

Drug Therapy for Hypertension

chapter 16

LEARNING ACTIVITIES

Matching

Match the correct mechanism of action on the right with its drug classification on the left.
(Answers will be used only once.)

_____ 1. Diuretic

_____ 2. Beta blocker

_____ 3. ACE inhibitor

_____ 4. Angiotensin II receptor agonist

_____ 5. Calcium channel blocker

_____ 6. Alpha blocker

_____ 7. Alpha-beta blocker

_____ 8. Central-acting adrenergic agent

_____ 9. Direct vasodilator

A. Combine alpha/beta blocker effects
B. Slow movement of calcium into cells
C. Oppose excitatory effects of norepinephrine at alpha receptors
D. Limit epinephrine activity
E. Stimulate brain alpha receptors
F. Eliminate salt and water from body
G. Cause arterial dilation
H. Block vasoconstrictors
I. Change action of renin-angiotensin-aldosterone system

Fill in the Blank

Fill in the blanks for each question with the correct answers.

10. Diffuse swelling of the face including the eyes, lips, and tongue is a characteristic of _____.

11. Beta blockers and alpha blockers affect the _____ receptors.

12. Hardening of the arterial walls is characteristic of _____.

13. Orthostatic hypotension manifests within 3 minutes of when a patient _____.

14. Secondary hypertension is related to specific _____ and _____.

MEDICATION SAFETY PRACTICE

____ 1.   A patient has forgotten to take a dose of prescribed medication for hypertension. What do you advise the patient to do?
A. Take double the amount when it is time for the next dose.
B. If the next dose is in less than 4 hours, just skip the dose that was missed.
C. Since the next dose is due in 2 hours, take the missed dose right away.
D. Take the missed dose immediately, and then skip the next scheduled dose.

____ 2.   As a result of reduced fluid volume and relaxation of arteries, most patients taking diuretics are at risk for which side effect?
A. Dehydration
B. Dizziness
C. Dementia
D. Demineralization

____ 3.   Stopping therapy with beta blockers should be done on what schedule?
A. Daily
B. Weekly
C. Gradually
D. Immediately

____ 4.   Captopril (Capoten) 25 mg PO is prescribed. The pharmacy sends scored tablets of 12.5 mg. How many tablets should be administered?
A. ½
B. 2
C. 2½
D. 4

____ 5.   What is your priority action for a patient who develops angioedema while taking angiotensin-converting enzyme (ACE) inhibitors?
A. Hold the next dose of medication to see if the condition improves.
B. Discontinue the medication and call the prescriber.
C. Administer the medication slowly and observe the patient's reaction.
D. Decrease the dose by one-half to see if the condition improves.

PRACTICE QUIZ

____ 1.   A patient is taking a calcium channel blocker. Which best describes how this medication lowers blood pressure?
A. It increases the movement of calcium into the cells of the heart and blood vessels.
B. It relaxes the body's blood vessels.
C. It decreases the supply of oxygen-rich blood to the heart.
D. It limits the activity of epinephrine on the heart and blood vessels.

____ 2.   A patient has been taking captopril (Capoten) for several weeks when severe swelling of the lips and difficulty breathing develop. This is recognized as which adverse effect?
A. Neutropenia
B. Photosensitivity
C. Reactive airway disease
D. Angioedema

____ 3. After administering losartan (Cozaar), the patient is monitored for which condition?
A. Potassium level higher than 5.5 mEq/L
B. Potassium level of 4.0 mEq/L
C. Decreased bowel sounds and constipation
D. Weight loss and increased urine output

____ 4. Which statement by a patient best indicates a correct understanding of instructions about taking angiotensin-converting enzyme (ACE) inhibitors?
A. "I'll use a salt substitute to flavor my food."
B. "After several months I won't need to worry about facial swelling."
C. "I'll need to use sunscreen and protective clothing for my trip to the beach."
D. "If I drink alcohol, my blood pressure would likely increase."

____ 5. Which statement about angiotensin-converting enzyme (ACE) inhibitors and pregnant women is true?
A. After delivery, ACE inhibitors can be used by a breastfeeding woman.
B. ACE inhibitors can cause liver disorders in the infant.
C. ACE inhibitors are category D drugs that can cause birth defects.
D. ACE inhibitors can cause the infant to develop hypokalemia.

____ 6. A patient who is taking atenolol (Tenormin), a beta blocker, should be monitored for which side effects? *(Select all that apply.)*
____ A. Tachycardia
____ B. Difficulty breathing
____ C. Fever or sore throat
____ D. Dizziness when standing up
____ E. Hyperkalemia

____ 7. A patient who has been taking a calcium channel blocker should be monitored for which symptoms of Stevens-Johnson syndrome?
A. Hypothermia
B. Gingival hyperplasia
C. Gynecomastia
D. Skin lesions

____ 8. Male patients who are taking which antihypertensive drug should be instructed not to take drugs for erectile dysfunction? *(Select all that apply.)*
____ A. Beta blockers
____ B. Alpha-beta blockers
____ C. Alpha blockers
____ D. Calcium channel blockers
____ E. DHT blockers

____ 9. Which drug has been safely used to treat pregnancy-induced hypertension?
A. Valsartan (Diovan)
B. Captopril (Capoten)
C. Methyldopa (Aldomet)
D. Atenolol (Tenormin)

____ 10. A patient who is taking losartan (Cozaar) is going on a 2-week cruise to the Bahamas during the summer. The patient should be advised to avoid which activities while on the cruise? *(Select all that apply.)*
____ A. Sitting for long periods of time
____ B. Consuming alcoholic beverages
____ C. Exercising on the boat deck
____ D. Eating fried or unusually spicy foods
____ E. Taking a drug to treat erectile dysfunction

____ 11. A patient who has been taking metoprolol (Lopressor) for several months states, "I've got nothing to live for any more. I'd be better off if I just died. I'm just depressed all the time." What should be the nurse's next action? *(Select all that apply.)*
____ A. Discuss the possibility of a dose increase with the prescriber.
____ B. Remind the patient of the importance of taking this medication.
____ C. Tell the patient to stop taking the medication immediately.
____ D. Inform the prescriber of the patient's possible depression symptoms.

_____ 12. A patient contacts the clinic at 4 PM on a Friday, saying she has just run out of the prescription for atenolol (Tenormin) which she takes for hypertension. The prescriber has left for the weekend, and the pharmacist will not refill the prescription without a refill authorization for the medication. What would be the nurse's best action?

A. Contact the on-call prescriber for a refill authorization.
B. Report the pharmacist to the state board of pharmacy.
C. Ask the patient to call the office back first thing Monday.
D. Ask the patient to remain calm.

Drug Therapy for Heart Failure

LEARNING ACTIVITIES

Fill in the Blank

Fill in the blanks with the correct answers.

1. For a headache related to initial treatment with nitroglycerin, the patient should take _____.

2. Heart failure is characterized by a dilated or overstretched _____ _____.

3. Decreased renal blood flow related to heart failure is compensated by activation of the _____ _____ _____.

4. Most heart failure begins in the _____ _____.

5. Digoxin increases the force of _____ _____.

Matching

Match the vasodilator on the left with the correct intended response on the right. (Not all options will be used, and some will be used more than once.)

_____ 6. hydralazine (Apresoline)

_____ 7. nitroglycerin

_____ 8. isosorbide (Isordil)

A. Decreased heart workload
B. Increased blood pressure
C. Increased blood flow to coronary arteries
D. Vasoconstriction of arteries
E. Increased venous vasodilation
F. Decreased blood pressure
G. Increased arterial vasodilation
H. Decreased blood flow to coronary arteries

Matching

Match the symptom of heart failure with the appropriate cause. (Answers will be used more than once.)

_____ 9. Shortness of breath

_____ 10. Oliguria during the day

_____ 11. Distended abdomen

_____ 12. Frothy, pink-tinged sputum

_____ 13. Crackles and wheezes

_____ 14. Enlarged liver

A. Right-sided heart failure

B. Left-sided heart failure

MEDICATION SAFETY PRACTICE

Determine whether each statement is True or False. If the statement is false, rewrite it to make it true.

_____ 1. Previous doses of nitroglycerin ointment should be vigorously rubbed off before administering a new dose.

_____ 2. Nitroglycerin ointment should be kept on the patient's skin around the clock in order to maintain a therapeutic blood level.

_____ 3. Digoxin (Lanoxin) toxicity may be characterized by bradycardia, loss of appetite, and yellow halos appearing around objects.

_____ 4. The trade name for the drug dopamine is Dobutamine.

Solve this problem:

5. Digoxin (Lanoxin) 0.25 mg PO is prescribed. The medication is available in scored tablets of 0.125 mg each. How should this dose be administered?

PRACTICE QUIZ

____ 1. A patient taking hydralazine (Apresoline) for heart failure has a temperature of 104° F. His white blood cell (WBC) count has dropped from 8000/mm³ to 4000/mm³. What is the patient at risk for experiencing?
A. Bleeding
B. Seizure
C. Infection
D. Falling

____ 2. A patient on digoxin (Lanoxin) reports feeling tired and nauseated. What is the priority assessment to make?
A. Temperature
B. Urine output
C. Apical pulse
D. Mental status

____ 3. Before administering nitroglycerin ointment to a patient, what precaution should be taken?
A. Putting on a facemask
B. Handwashing with bactericidal solution
C. Putting on a gown
D. Putting on gloves

____ 4. Which instruction should be given to the patient regarding oral nitroglycerin?
A. "Keep it in the refrigerator."
B. "Store the amber bottle in a dark place."
C. "Keep a drink of water close by so you can swallow the pills quickly in an emergency."
D. "If you do not feel a tingling sensation, the drug is no longer potent."

____ 5. Female patients of childbearing age who are or may become pregnant should be told what about taking digoxin (Lanoxin)?
A. "Drink plenty of water before breastfeeding."
B. "Digoxin passes from the mother to the fetus."
C. "This drug is perfectly safe for your baby."
D. "Try to exercise regularly to reduce the drug's effect on the fetus."

____ 6. Hydralazine (Apresoline) dosage in children is based on what measurement?
A. Height
B. Age
C. Heart rate
D. Weight

____ 7. What is the correct initial dose of nesiritide (Natrecor) for an adult who weighs 68 kg in heart failure?
A. 10 mcg
B. 130 mcg
C. 136 mcg
D. 100 mcg

____ 8. After beginning therapy with IV potassium for heart failure, a patient's cardiac monitor shows an irregular heart rate of 60 beats per minute. The patient reports feeling weak and confused. The prescriber is notified if the patient's serum potassium is in what range (expressed in mmol/L)?
A. 3.5-5.0
B. 1.5-3.0
C. 0.5-1.5
D. 5.2-6.8

____ 9. Which instruction should be included when teaching a patient about the use of digoxin (Lanoxin)?
A. "If this medication causes an upset stomach, take it with an antacid."
B. "Take your pulse monthly and notify your prescriber if your pulse is less than 60."
C. "Digoxin toxicity is less likely to occur if you are also taking diuretics."
D. "Keep all laboratory appointments for drug level testing."

____ 10. A patient is undergoing treatment for heart failure with dopamine. Which is a possible side effect of this treatment?
A. The cardiac output is increased.
B. The heart rate lowers 20 beats per minute.
C. The white blood cell count is lowered.
D. Tissue damage occurs if there is infiltration.

11. A patient has received instructions on increasing potassium intake in the diet. The patient demonstrates understanding of the instructions by selecting which menu items? *(Select all that apply.)*

_____ A.   Tuna sandwich

_____ B.   Baked potato

_____ C.   Brazil nuts

_____ D.   Winter squash

_____ E.   Black beans

Drug Therapy for Dysrhythmias

chapter
18

LEARNING ACTIVITIES

Matching

Match the drug on the left with its correct drug category on the right. (Answers will be used more than once.)

_____ 1. lidocaine (Xylocaine)

_____ 2. esmolol (Brevibloc)

_____ 3. tocainide (Tonocard)

_____ 4. propranolol (Inderal)

_____ 5. amiodarone (Cordarone)

_____ 6. diltiazem (Cardizem)

_____ 7. verapamil (Calan)

A. Beta blocker
B. Potassium channel blocker
C. Calcium channel blocker
D. Class 1b sodium channel blocker

Fill in the Blank

Fill in the blanks with the correct answers.

8. The ability of the cardiac muscle cells to fire on their own is known as

_____.

9. Before administering atropine (Atropine Sulfate), the nurse must assess for a history of _____.

10. To treat digoxin toxicity, a drug is given to bind with the medication and prevent its action. The generic and trade names of this drug are _____ and _____.

List the medications which may be given through the endotracheal tube during a cardiac/ respiratory emergency when an intravenous line has not been established.

11. _____

12. _____

13. _____

14. _____

15. _____

MEDICATION SAFETY PRACTICE

1. Some of the life-threatening effects of procainamide are
    _____, _____, _____,
    and _____.

2. Some serious adverse effects of dofetilide (Tikosyn) are
    _____ and _____.

3. In addition to signs of thyroid problems, what should a patient taking amiodarone (Cordarone) be monitored for?

    _____

    _____

4. A health care professional is administering adenosine (Adenocard). What special injection technique is required?

5. The patient who is taking amiodarone (Cordarone) is instructed to have eye examinations every 6 to 12 months to assess for _____
    _____.

PRACTICE QUIZ

_____ 1. Before beginning treatment with atropine (Atropine Sulfate) for bradycardia, the nurse should assess for a history of which disorder in the patient?
    A. Multiple sclerosis
    B. Muscular dystrophy
    C. Glaucoma
    D. Diabetes

_____ 2. What is the correct dose in milligrams of quinidine (Quinidine Sulfate) for a 3-year-old child who weighs 22 pounds?
    A. 16
    B. 25
    C. 37
    D. 60

_____ 3. A patient taking digoxin (Lanoxin) reports a weight gain of 7 pounds in the last week. The nurse should assess the patient for the possibility of which condition?
    A. Pregnancy
    B. Clinical depression
    C. Bowel obstruction
    D. Heart failure

_____ 4. In an emergency, lidocaine (Xylocaine) may be given intravenously or by airway inhalation. Why are these routes of administration used?
    A. They avoid interaction with other drugs.
    B. They reduce the risk of adverse effects.
    C. When given orally, the liver renders the drug ineffective.
    D. They are closer to the tissue where drug action is needed most.

_____ 5. Patients who are taking tocainide (Tonocard) may have increased risk of infection because of what adverse effect?
    A. Pneumonitis
    B. Confusion
    C. Neutropenia
    D. Hypotension

6. Which drugs are used to treat ventricular dysrhythmias? *(Select all that apply.)*
   ____ A.   atropine (Atropine Sulfate)
   ____ B.   lidocaine (Xylocaine)
   ____ C.   digoxin (Lanoxin)
   ____ D.   flecainide (Tambocor)
   ____ E.   digoxin immune fab (DigiFab)
   ____ F.   propranolol (Inderal)
   ____ G.   esmolol (Brevibloc)

____ 7. A patient is experiencing bradycardia accompanied by symptoms of dizziness. Which medication is most likely to be prescribed for this patient?
   A.   Adenosine
   B.   Atropine
   C.   Amiodarone
   D.   Atenolol

8. What is the correct dose in milligrams of ibutilide (Corvert) for an adult patient who weighs 140 pounds? (The recommended adult dose for a patient weighing less than 60 kg is 0.01 mg/kg over 1 minute; 1 mg for a patient over 60 kg.)
   _____ mg

9. An older adult has been given a dose of lidocaine (Xylocaine). Which interventions are important to include? *(Select all that apply.)*
   ____ A.   Instruct the patient to change positions slowly.
   ____ B.   Advise the patient to use handrails to reduce the risk for falls.
   ____ C.   Advise the patient to report episodes of diarrhea.
   ____ D.   Monitor laboratory results for increased white blood cells.
   ____ E.   Observe the patient for episodes of confusion.

____ 10. A patient who has been taking amiodarone (Cordarone) for several months mentions difficulty breathing and a cough, which has been present for several weeks. Which action is most appropriate?
   A.   Report the patient's symptoms to the health care provider.
   B.   Suggest screening for the possibility of tuberculosis infection.
   C.   Advise the patient these are common and expected side effects.
   D.   Teach the patient these side effects usually resolve with time.

____ 11. A patient who has been taking amiodarone (Cordarone) for several months is discussing a trip to the American southwest during May and June. Which recommendation is most important?
   A.   Restrict liquid intake and minimize exposure to heat.
   B.   It would be better if you stayed at home instead of vacationing.
   C.   Wear dark sunglasses and protective clothing when outdoors.
   D.   Ask your provider to temporarily stop the amiodarone while on the trip.

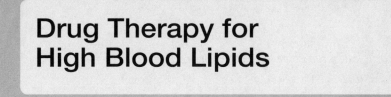

Drug Therapy for High Blood Lipids

chapter
19

LEARNING ACTIVITIES

Crossword Puzzle: Lipid-Lowering Drugs

Complete the puzzle by identifying the correct terms that are described.

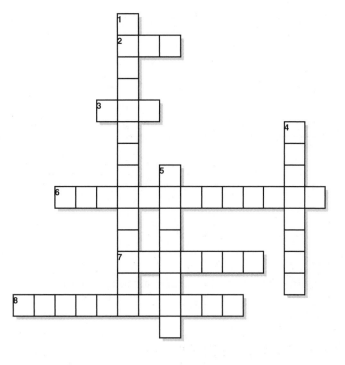

Across
2. "Good" cholesterol in the body (abbreviation)
3. "Bad" cholesterol in the body (abbreviation)
6. Vitamin B that helps decrease cholesterol levels (two words)
7. Drugs that inhibit production of cholesterol
8. Waxy, fatty material in cell walls

Down
1. Muscle cell breakdown
4. Genetic hyperlipidemia
5. Drugs that lower triglycerides

Matching

Match the drug with its appropriate drug category. (Some drug categories will be used more than once.)

____ 1.   atorvastatin (Lipitor)

____ 2.   ezetimibe (Zetia)

____ 3.   niacin extended release (Niaspan)

____ 4.   pravastatin (Pravachol)

____ 5.   cholestyramine (Questran)

____ 6.   gemfibrozil (Lopid)

____ 7.   fenofibrate (Tricor)

____ 8.   colestipol (Colestid)

____ 9.   simvastatin (Zocor)

A. Bile acid sequestrant
B. Cholesterol absorption inhibitor
C. Fibrate
D. Nicotinic acid
E. Statin

Fill in the Blank

Fill in the blanks with the correct answers.

10. The side effect of flushing or hot flashes when taking nicotinic acid (Niacor) can be reduced by taking the drug with _____ or with _____.

11. Patients with diabetes must be taught that nicotinic acid (Niacor) can have the effect of _____ blood glucose levels.

12. Bile acid sequestrant drugs bind cholesterol-containing bile in the _____ and remove them via _____ _____.

13. Cholesterol absorption inhibitors prevent the uptake of cholesterol from the _____ _____ into the _____ _____.

14. _____ primarily lower triglycerides.

15. Statin drugs lower LDL cholesterol and triglycerides by _____ _____ by the body.

MEDICATION SAFETY PRACTICE

1. Before beginning therapy with lipid-lowering drugs, the patient must have baseline testing done for _____ function.

2. Statins should not be given to patients who drink more than _____ alcoholic beverages a day.

3. Fibrates can increase the effectiveness of warfarin (Coumadin) and cause a prolonged _____ time.

4. Gemfibrozil (Lopid) may interact with statin drugs by interfering with their _____.

5. A patient has been taking rosuvastatin (Crestor) for several months to lower the cholesterol level. Today the patient mentions having abdominal pain under the ribs on the right side and having darker urine and lighter gray stools. What is the likely explanation for this?

    _____

    _____

6. In the above situation, what should be the next action?

    _____

    _____

PRACTICE QUIZ

1. What lifestyle changes are discussed with a patient who is beginning drug therapy for treatment of hyperlipidemia and hypercholesterolemia? *(Select all that apply.)*
   - ____ A. Weight control
   - ____ B. Ergonomic workstation
   - ____ C. Regular exercise
   - ____ D. Driving at night
   - ____ E. Low-fat diet
   - ____ F. Organic diet

2. Although generally safe for older adults, which conditions are contraindications for medication therapy with statins? *(Select all that apply.)*
   - ____ A. Diabetes mellitus
   - ____ B. Glaucoma
   - ____ C. Liver disease
   - ____ D. Hypertension
   - ____ E. Myopathy
   - ____ F. Alzheimer's disease

____ 3. The patient is instructed to take the tablet form of bile acid sequestrants with at least how many ounces of water?
   - A. 2-4
   - B. 6-9
   - C. 10-12
   - D. 12-16

____ 4. What beverage interferes with the metabolism of fibrates and makes them less effective?
   - A. Coffee
   - B. Milk
   - C. Grapefruit juice
   - D. Pomegranate juice

5. A patient has been taking nicotinic acid (Niacor) for several months and is now at a dosage of 1 g twice per day. The medication is available in 500-mg tablets. How many tablets per day will the patient take? _____ tablet(s)

____ 6. Which intervention can reduce the flushing or hot flashes associated with nicotinic acid?
   - A. Give the drug with estrogen hormone replacement.
   - B. Administer the drug with acetaminophen (Tylenol).
   - C. Give the drug with large amounts of fluid.
   - D. Give the drug during or after a full meal.

_____ 7. A patient who is taking a statin agent should be monitored for which serious adverse effect?
   A. Decreased liver function
   B. Decreased platelet counts
   C. Increased white blood cell counts
   D. Hypotension and tachycardia

_____ 8. A patient asks how statin drugs work in the body. What is the best response?
   A. "They bind with cholesterol in the intestine."
   B. "They work by controlling the rate of cholesterol produced by the liver."
   C. "They reduce the amount of cholesterol absorbed by the body."
   D. "They are a type of vitamin B that increases HDL cholesterol."

_____ 9. An older adult taking a statin agent reports suddenly developing muscle aches and weakness. What is the most important question to ask this patient?
   A. "Have you taken any over-the-counter NSAIDs?"
   B. "Have you noticed any numbness or tingling sensations in your extremities?"
   C. "Have you noticed a brownish color to your urine?"
   D. "Have you noticed any facial flushing or 'hot flashes'?"

_____ 10. A patient's medication history is carefully reviewed by members of the health care team. The patient is currently taking warfarin (Coumadin). It is not likely this patient will have a bile acid sequestrant prescribed for which reason?
   A. The bile acid sequestrant would intensify the effect of warfarin.
   B. The bile acid sequestrant needs to be taken with aspirin.
   C. The bile acid sequestrant would cause the warfarin to be ineffective.
   D. The bile acid sequestrant would lower the overall platelet count.

_____ 11. A patient who will be taking gemfibrozil (Lopid) will be evaluated for which disorder as a possible adverse effect of the drug?
   A. Kidney stones
   B. Deep vein thrombosis
   C. Increased creatinine levels
   D. Constipation

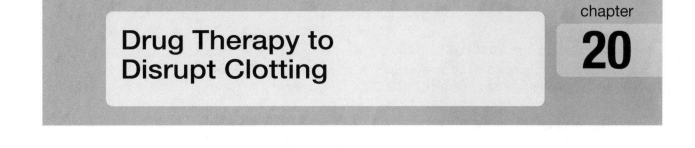

Drug Therapy to Disrupt Clotting

chapter

20

LEARNING ACTIVITIES

Crossword Puzzle: Terminology Review

Complete the puzzle by identifying the correct terms that are described.

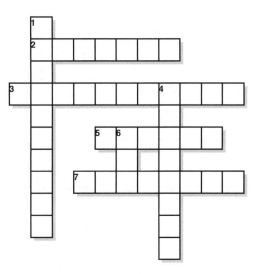

Across
2. Travels through the bloodstream and blocks vessels
3. Process by which blood clots form
5. Protein essence of a blood clot
7. Blood clot in a vessel or the heart

Down
1. Profuse bleeding
4. Converts fibrinogen to fibrin
6. Blood test used to report results of warfarin anticoagulation (abbreviation)

Matching

Match the type of anticoagulant drug on the right with the correct medication names on the left. (Answers will be used more than once.)

_____	1.	darbepoetin alfa (Aranesp)
_____	2.	warfarin (Coumadin)
_____	3.	ticlopidine (Ticlid)
_____	4.	t-PA (Activase)
_____	5.	clopidogrel (Plavix)
_____	6.	tenecteplase (TNKase)
_____	7.	tirofiban (Aggrastat)
_____	8.	reteplase (Retavase)
_____	9.	epoetin alfa (Epogen, Procrit)
_____	10.	eptifibatide (Integrilin)
_____	11.	heparin
_____	12.	oprelvekin (Neumega)
_____	13.	aspirin
_____	14.	enoxaparin (Lovenox)

A. Thrombin inhibitor
B. Clotting factor synthesis inhibitor
C. Antiplatelet
D. Thrombolytic
E. Colony-stimulating factor

Fill in the Blank

15. Clotting factor synthesis inhibitors decrease the production of clotting factors in the _____.

16. _____ drugs break down fibrin in an already-formed clot.

17. Thrombin inhibitors block the action of _____, which converts _____ to _____ to form clots.

18. _____ are drugs that interfere with blood clotting by preventing the activation of platelets.

19. _____ combine with proteins in the plasma to stick together and form a clot.

MEDICATION SAFETY PRACTICE

1. The recommended dose of oprelvekin (Neumega) is 50 mcg/kg once daily. The correct dose of this drug for an adult who weighs 154 pounds is _____ mcg.

2. Vitamin K is the antidote for _____.

3. Rubbing the injection site after administering subcutaneous heparin is likely to cause _____.

4. Colony-stimulating factors increase the patient's risk for hypertension, blood clots, strokes, and heart attacks because of increased blood _____ and _____ retention.

5. When a patient is taking an anticoagulant medication, a careful medication history review is completed. Which over-the-counter and herbal medications could cause additional bleeding?

6. A patient who is pregnant has a venous thromboembolism. Which medication will most likely be prescribed?

PRACTICE QUIZ

1. Which statement best demonstrates a patient's understanding of how warfarin (Coumadin) works to help after heart valve replacement surgery? *(Select all that apply.)*
   ____ A. "It will thin out my blood so that it won't clot anymore."
   ____ B. "It will make me bruise and bleed more easily, so I must be careful."
   ____ C. "It will dissolve the clots that have formed in my heart."
   ____ D. "New clots will not form as easily in my heart valves."
   ____ E. "Any clots that I still have will not get any bigger."
   ____ F. "I will feel the cold weather more because my blood is thinner now."

____ 2. Which lab tests are used to monitor the effectiveness of heparin administration to a patient who has had a venous thromboembolism (VTE)?
   A. Prothrombin time (PT)
   B. Activated partial prothrombin time (APPT)
   C. Activated partial thromboplastin time (aPTT)
   D. International normalized ratio (INR)

3. A patient who is taking warfarin (Coumadin) therapy is instructed to avoid which foods? *(Select all that apply.)*
   ____ A. Grapefruit
   ____ B. Fava beans
   ____ C. Spinach
   ____ D. Bananas
   ____ E. Kale
   ____ F. Oranges
   ____ G. Broccoli

____ 4. A patient on renal dialysis who is anemic is most likely to be administered which medication?
   A. Oprelvekin (Neumega)
   B. Alteplase/t-PA (Activase)
   C. Clopidogrel (Plavix)
   D. Epoetin alfa (Epogen, Procrit)

____ 5. A patient who is taking a clotting factor synthesis inhibitor such as warfarin (Coumadin) should be monitored for which serious adverse effect?
   A. Decreased clotting times
   B. Upset stomach, diarrhea, and fever
   C. Headaches that are severe and will not go away
   D. Increased viscosity of the blood

6. What are important lifespan considerations for an older adult who is taking warfarin (Coumadin)? *(Select all that apply.)*
   ____ A. Aspirin increases the action of warfarin.
   ____ B. Statin drugs decrease the action of warfarin.
   ____ C. Older adults are more likely to develop bruises and bleeding.
   ____ D. Sucralfate (Carafate) increases the effect of warfarin.
   ____ E. Older adults need more frequent monitoring of the international normalized ratio (INR).

____ 7. Which important instruction should be included when teaching patients about colony-stimulating factor therapy?
   A. Tell the patient that weight gain of more than 2 pounds a month should be reported to the prescriber.
   B. Teach the patient how to administer intramuscular injections correctly.
   C. Remind the patient to keep scheduled laboratory appointments for blood tests to monitor therapy.
   D. Instruct the patient to take this medication with adequate amounts of liquid.

____ 8. Several patients are receiving heparin. Which medication must be available on the unit to use as an antidote?
   A. Epoetin alfa (Epogen)
   B. Enoxaparin (Lovenox)
   C. Vitamin K (AquaMEPHYTON)
   D. Protamine sulfate

____ 9. Before administering a thrombolytic drug, the nurse assesses for which absolute contraindication?
   A. Chronic peptic ulcer disease
   B. Recent spinal or cerebral surgery
   C. Blood pressure of 150/92 mm Hg
   D. Current use of warfarin (Coumadin) or aspirin

____ 10. Diet instructions have been provided to a patient who will be taking warfarin (Coumadin) for several weeks. Which menu selection indicates the need for further instructions?
   A. Spinach salad with bacon dressing
   B. Orange and banana fruit salad
   C. Plate of assorted cheeses and grapes
   D. Pepperoni pizza and light beer

____ 11. A patient has recently been given an intravenous injection of heparin. Which vital sign changes should be reported as signs of a hemorrhage?
   A. Increased blood pressure, decreased pulse
   B. Decreased blood pressure, increased pulse
   C. Decreased blood pressure, decreased pulse
   D. Increased blood pressure, increased pulse

Drug Therapy for Asthma, Chronic Obstructive Pulmonary Disease, and Pulmonary Fibrosis/Hypertension

LEARNING ACTIVITIES

Matching

Match the correct drug category on the right with the correct medication names on the left. (Answers will be used more than once.)

____ 1. beclomethasone (QVAR)

____ 2. albuterol (Proventil)

____ 3. theophylline (Theo-Dur)

____ 4. triamcinolone (Azmacort)

____ 5. salmeterol (Serevent)

____ 6. fluticasone (Flovent)

____ 7. aminophylline (Truphylline)

____ 8. ipratropium (Atrovent)

____ 9. budesonide (Pulmicort)

____ 10. formoterol (Foradil)

____ 11. terbutaline (Brethine)

____ 12. cromolyn sodium (Intal)

____ 13. tiotropium (Spiriva)

____ 14. montelukast sodium (Singulair)

____ 15. nedocromil sodium (Tilade)

____ 16. zafirlukast (Accolate)

A. Short-acting beta$_2$ agonist
B. Long-acting beta$_2$ agonist
C. Cholinergic antagonist
D. Methylxanthine
E. Inhaled corticosteroid
F. Mast cell stabilizer
G. Leukotriene inhibitor

Terminology Review

Match the term on the right with its correct description on the left. (Answers will be used only once.)

_____ 17. Air sacs in the lungs where oxygen moves into the blood

_____ 18. Airway obstruction disease caused by constriction and inflammation

_____ 19. Sound of air moving through narrowed airways

_____ 20. Drug that reduces the thickness of mucus

_____ 21. Open center of a hollow airway

_____ 22. Inflammation of the airways

_____ 23. Disease where the elasticity of alveoli is greatly reduced

_____ 24. Tightening of pulmonary smooth muscle, resulting in narrowed airways

_____ 25. Drug that relaxes the smooth muscle around airways, causing the center openings to enlarge

A. Lumen
B. Alveoli
C. Bronchitis
D. Asthma
E. Mucolytic
F. Emphysema
G. Wheeze
H. Bronchodilator
I. Bronchoconstriction

Matching: Pathophysiology of Asthma and COPD

Indicate which characteristics are associated only with asthma, which are associated only with COPD, and which are common to both. (Answers will be used more than once.)

_____ 26. Involves the airways and the alveoli

_____ 27. Causes reduced oxygenation

_____ 28. Is a reversible condition of airway obstruction

_____ 29. Wheezing

_____ 30. Increased size of mucus-producing cells

_____ 31. Caused by a combination of bronchitis and emphysema

_____ 32. Reduces peak expiratory flow rate (PEFR)

_____ 33. No symptoms present between attacks

_____ 34. Lumen size is reduced

_____ 35. Can be caused by constriction of bronchiolar smooth muscle alone

_____ 36. Airway inflammation

_____ 37. Loss of elastic tissue in walls of the alveoli

A. Asthma
B. COPD
C. Both

Fill in the Blank

38. A common method to measure airway function is _____

    _____ _____

    _____ (_____).

39. A patient can use a(n) _____ _____
    when about to start an activity that is likely to induce an asthma attack.

40. List four systemic effects of bronchodilators. _____

    _____

    _____

41. _____ or _____ _____ can occur if excessive amounts of bronchodilator drugs reach the blood.

42. A child who takes a(n) _____ _____ _____ close to bedtime may have difficulty sleeping.

MEDICATION SAFETY PRACTICE

1. Asthma medication that is used only during an acute episode is known as a(n) _____ drug.

2. A patient just took a short-acting inhaler drug. What symptoms of an adverse effect should be reported immediately to the prescriber?

3. The nurse must ensure that the patient using an oral inhaler knows the proper technique for using it, and for a(n) _____, if one is ordered.

4. If a patient is taking more than one type of inhaled drug, the _____ drug should be given at least 5 minutes before the other drug.

5. A PEFR value that has dropped below 50% indicates what is occurring?

PRACTICE QUIZ

_____ 1. Symptom severity in a patient with asthma or chronic bronchitis is assessed by using which method?
A. FEV_1
B. PEFR
C. PEEP
D. CPAP

_____ 2. A patient is taking ipratropium (Atrovent), and reports having difficulty emptying his bladder. What should be the nurse's action?
A. Report symptoms of kidney disease to the prescriber.
B. Encourage the patient to drink more fluids.
C. Ask the prescriber for an order for an indwelling catheter.
D. Discuss the patient's symptoms with the prescriber.

_____ 3. Which important point should be included when teaching patients about the use of long-acting beta$_2$-adrenergic agonists?
A. "Use this medication whenever you have new symptoms of wheezing."
B. "Take an extra dose of this medication if your symptoms worsen."
C. "Take this medication even when symptoms are not present."
D. "Omit your daily dose of this medication if you are wheezing."

_____ 4. A child with asthma is having difficulty using a "rescue" aerosol inhaler effectively. What alteration in treatment should be discussed with the provider?
A. Switching the route of administration to oral
B. Using a nebulized form of the drug with a facemask
C. Switching to a dry powder inhaler
D. Changing to a long-acting inhaler

5. What are common side effects associated with inhaled anti-inflammatory drugs? *(Select all that apply.)*
   ____ A. Bad taste
   ____ B. Mouth dryness
   ____ C. Seizures
   ____ D. Leukopenia
   ____ E. Oral infection

____ 6. Before administering an inhaled corticosteroid, it is important to take which action?
   A. Teach the patient how to use the inhaler or spacer.
   B. Teach the patient to expect nervousness after using.
   C. Prime a new canister of nedocromil (Tilade) once before use.
   D. Administer inhaled corticosteroid agents before bronchodilators.

____ 7. What important instruction should be given to a patient who is taking guaifenesin (Mucinex)?
   A. "This medication is given to treat acetaminophen overdose."
   B. "This medication will thin your mucus and make it easier to cough up."
   C. "This medication can cause an oral infection called *thrush*."
   D. "This medication is used with a nebulizer facemask."

____ 8. A patient has just taken a short-acting inhaler drug to treat asthma symptoms. Which best indicates the medication has been effective?
   A. An increase in the respiratory rate
   B. A pulse oximetry value of 85%
   C. An increase of 15% in the peak flow
   D. Wheezing within 2 hours of use

____ 9. A patient has been given instructions on use of a dry-powder inhaler. Which patient action indicates the need for further instructions?
   A. The patient exhales deeply into the inhaler after the treatment.
   B. The patient stores the device in a dry place, at room temperature.
   C. The patient states she knows not to shake the inhaler prior to use.
   D. The patient removes the inhaler from her mouth as soon as she has inhaled.

____ 10. A patient is using an aerosol inhaler without a spacer. Two puffs are prescribed. How far apart should the puffs be administered?
   A. 10 seconds
   B. 30 seconds
   C. 60 seconds
   D. 120 seconds

____ 11. Which action by the nurse is most essential during intravenous administration of treprostinil (Orenitram) for a patient with pulmonary hypertension?
   A. Disconnect the intravenous line when assisting the patient to the bathroom.
   B. Utilize strict sterile technique when preparing and administering the drug.
   C. Connect intravenous antibiotic drugs to the same line to prevent needle pain.
   D. Monitor the patient's laboratory tests for signs of deteriorating kidney function.

____ 12. Which is the most important point to include in patient teaching for a female patient with pulmonary hypertension who will have bosentan (Tracleer) prescribed?
   A. "We can electronically transfer this prescription to your retail pharmacist."
   B. "A yellowish tinge to your skin is common while taking this medication."
   C. "If you have any difficulty swallowing the tablet, cut it in half."
   D. "Your pregnancy test must be negative before this drug can be given."

Drug Therapy for Gastrointestinal Dysfunction

chapter

22

LEARNING ACTIVITIES

Terminology Review

Match the definitions on the right with their correct terms on the left. (Answers will be used only once.)

_____ 1. Antiemetic

_____ 2. Chemoreceptor

_____ 3. Constipation

_____ 4. Diarrhea

_____ 5. Emesis

_____ 6. Mechanoreceptors

_____ 7. Nausea

_____ 8. Peristalsis

_____ 9. Retching

_____ 10. Vestibular apparatus

_____ 11. Vomiting

A. Frequent watery bowel movements
B. Act or results of vomiting
C. Tension receptors in the bowel that initiate vomiting
D. Forcing stomach contents up through the esophagus and out of the mouth
E. Urge to vomit
F. Labored respiration with the contraction of the abdomen, chest wall, and diaphragm
G. Sensory nerve cells responding to intestinal chemical stimuli and toxins
H. Inner ear structures associated with balance and position sensing
I. Bowel movements that are infrequent and difficult or painful
J. Mass movements in the colon
K. Drugs that prevent or control nausea

Matching

Match the drug category on the right with the correct drug names on the left. (Answers will be used more than once.)

_____ 12. docusate (Colace)

_____ 13. loperamide (Imodium)

_____ 14. prochlorperazine (Compazine)

_____ 15. bismuth subsalicylate (Pepto-Bismol)

_____ 16. meclizine (Dramamine)

_____ 17. difenoxin with atropine (Motofen)

_____ 18. lactulose (Cephulac)

_____ 19. diphenoxylate with atropine (Lomotil)

_____ 20. bisacodyl (Dulcolax)

_____ 21. calcium polycarbophil (FiberCon)

_____ 22. scopolamine (L-hyoscine)

_____ 23. granisetron (Kytril)

_____ 24. metoclopramide (Reglan)

_____ 25. castor oil (Emulsoil)

A. Antidiarrheal drug
B. Antiemetic drug
C. Drug for constipation

Matching: Drugs for Nausea and Vomiting

Match the type of action with the corresponding antiemetic drug. (Each answer will be used only once.)

_____ 26. Block dopamine receptors to inhibit one or more vomiting reflex pathways

_____ 27. Inhibit vomiting reflex pathways to stop intestinal cramping and inhibit vestibular input

_____ 28. Block the action of histamine at the H_1 receptor sites, which results in depression of inner ear excitability and reduces vestibular excitability

_____ 29. Bind to and block serotonin receptors in the intestinal tract, which results in blockage of at least two pathways of the vomiting reflex

_____ 30. Directly block dopamine from binding to receptors in the chemotrigger zone and the intestinal tract so that food moves along the intestinal tract more rapidly

A. Dopamine antagonists
B. Antihistamines
C. 5HT3-receptor antagonists
D. Anticholinergics
E. Phenothiazines

Fill in the Blank

31. A(n) _____ drug treats diarrhea by slowing down peristalsis in the gastrointestinal tract.

32. A dopamine antagonist binds to receptors in the _____ _____.

33. A lubricant is a(n) _____ or _____ substance that can help make bowel movements easier.

34. By adding fluid to stool, _____ _____ make bowel movements easier.

35. An antihistamine drug works against nausea/vomiting by blocking the action of histamine at the _____ _____ _____.

36. _____ _____ _____ are drugs that work against nausea and vomiting caused by chemotherapy treatments.

MEDICATION SAFETY PRACTICE

1. A patient is to receive 35 mg of promethazine (Phenergan) IM. The vial that is available contains 50 mg/mL. How much promethazine will be given to the patient? _____ mL

2. List three causes of constipation.

3. List five symptoms of neuroleptic malignant syndrome.

4. A patient who lives in a hot, humid environment should be advised that taking an antinausea drug such as _____ can cause anticholinergic effects leading to a decrease in sweating, and an increased risk of overheating the body.

5. List three symptoms of Reye's syndrome.

PRACTICE QUIZ

_____ 1. Which drug is likely to be most helpful in controlling nausea and vomiting in a patient receiving chemotherapy?
A. Metoclopramide (Reglan)
B. Trimethobenzamide (Tigan)
C. Scopolamine (L-hyoscine)
D. Ondansetron (Zofran)

_____ 2. Which drug for the control of nausea and vomiting is contraindicated in a patient who has a history of depression?
A. Promethazine (Phenergan)
B. Prochlorperazine (Compazine)
C. Scopolamine (L-hyoscine)
D. Metoclopramide (Reglan)

_____ 3. After continued administration of promethazine (Phenergan) or prochlorperazine (Compazine), which laboratory result needs to be monitored?
A. Blood urea nitrogen (BUN)
B. Complete blood count (CBC)
C. International normalized ratio (INR)
D. Activated partial thromboplastin time (aPTT)

_____ 4. An older adult woman who has problems with constipation wants to know which drug is safe for her to take on a daily or alternate-day schedule. Which drug will most likely be recommended by the health care provider?
A. Polyethylene glycol (MiraLax)
B. Castor oil (Emulsoil)
C. Sodium phosphate (Fleet Enema)
D. Psyllium (Metamucil)

_____ 5. A patient with diabetes is advised to take a laxative every other day if no bowel movement occurs. Which laxative is contraindicated for this patient?
A. Bisacodyl (Dulcolax)
B. Lactulose (Cephulac)
C. Polyethylene glycol (MiraLax)
D. Magnesium hydroxide (Milk of Magnesia)

6. An older adult who is taking an antiemetic drug requires additional monitoring for which side effects? _(Select all that apply.)_
_____ A. Confusion
_____ B. Shuffling gait
_____ C. Diarrhea
_____ D. Excessive drooling
_____ E. Trembling

_____ 7. Which statement indicates the patient has understood how to achieve the best response from medications for chemotherapy-induced nausea?
A. "I will take an antiemetic medication 30 minutes before meals."
B. "I will take this medication every night with a small glass of wine."
C. "I will take this medication within 1 hour after chemotherapy begins."
D. "The lip-smacking and tongue movements I am experiencing are expected effects."

_____ 8. After administering a medication for diarrhea to a patient, what is most important to do?
A. Instruct the patient to restrict oral fluids.
B. Remind the patient to decrease his or her activity level.
C. Assess the patient for abdominal distention.
D. Assess the patient's fasting blood sugar.

9. A patient who experiences toxic megacolon after taking antimotility drugs would exhibit which signs and symptoms? _(Select all that apply.)_
_____ A. Bradycardia
_____ B. Fever
_____ C. Abdominal pain
_____ D. Distended abdomen
_____ E. Hypervolemia

____ 10. A patient is very nauseated after surgery. What is a very dangerous direct complication of this?
  A. Increased risk for aspiration pneumonia
  B. Increased risk for fluid volume overload
  C. Excessive scar tissue from surgical incision
  D. Risk for development of venous thromboembolism

____ 11. A patient is undergoing chemotherapy and has been experiencing nausea and vomiting with each session. Which instruction is most likely to help prevent future nausea events?
  A. "Avoid chemotherapy treatments due to the severity of nausea and vomiting."
  B. "Take the prescribed antiemetic prior to arrival for chemotherapy treatments."
  C. "Let us know once you become nauseated, so we can give you antiemetic medication."
  D. "Nausea and vomiting are seldom associated with chemotherapy treatments."

____ 12. A patient who frequently experiences motion sickness will be taking meclizine (Antivert) prior to airplane travel. The patient should be instructed that which side effect is common with the medication?
  A. Constipation
  B. Involuntary muscle movements
  C. Drowsiness
  D. Abdominal pain

Drug Therapy for Gastric Ulcers and Reflux

LEARNING ACTIVITIES

Terminology Review

Match each description on the right with its correct term on the left. (Answers will be used only once.)

_____ 1. Antacids
_____ 2. Barrett's esophagus
_____ 3. Dyspepsia
_____ 4. Lower esophageal sphincter (LES)
_____ 5. Esophagogastroduodenoscopy (EGD)
_____ 6. Gastroesophageal reflux disease (GERD)
_____ 7. Gastric ulcer
_____ 8. *Helicobacter pylori*
_____ 9. H$_2$ blocker
_____ 10. Peritonitis
_____ 11. Regurgitation

A. Indigestion
B. Open sore in the stomach lining
C. Upper endoscopy exam of the esophagus, stomach, and small intestine
D. Complication of severe chronic GERD
E. Esophageal irritation due to stomach acid backing up
F. Drugs that block the effects of histamine
G. Backward flow of stomach contents
H. Inflammation of the abdominal cavity
I. Bacteria that cause gastric inflammation
J. Drugs that neutralize stomach acids
K. Muscular ring located where the esophagus joins the stomach

Multiple Choice

_____ 12. What percentage of people in the U.S. develop an ulcer during their lifetime?
   A. 5%
   B. 10%
   C. 15%
   D. 20%

_____ 13. Of the following causes of gastric ulcers, which one is primary?
   A. Stress
   B. Diet
   C. Excess gastric acid
   D. *H. pylori*

_____ 14. Which weakened sphincter muscle causes GERD?
   A. Anal
   B. Upper esophageal
   C. Pyloric
   D. Lower esophageal

15. Which dietary factors contribute to reflux? *(Select all that apply.)*

____ A.   Caffeine

____ B.   Nicotine

____ C.   Chewing gum

____ D.   Chocolate

____ E.   Black pepper

____ F.   Alcohol

____ G.   Red meats

____ H.   Peppermint

____ I.   Small meals

____ J.   Leafy green vegetables

____ K.   Eggs

Fill in the Blank

16. When _____ _____ exceeds mucus production, the risk for ulcers increases.

17. List four symptoms of a gastric ulcer. _____

_____

_____

_____

18. Usually, the pain of a peptic ulcer is located between the _____ and _____.

19. _____ _____ after a meal may prevent irritation of the esophagus associated with GERD.

20. Chronic GERD can lead to serious complications such as _____ _____ and _____ _____.

Matching: Types of Drugs for PUD and GERD

Match the type of drug used for peptic ulcer disease (PUD) and GERD with its action. (Each answer will be used only once.)

____ 21.   Decrease the secretion of gastric acid

____ 22.   Block the secretion of gastric acid

____ 23.   Form a thick coating that covers an ulcer to protect it from further damage

____ 24.   Neutralize stomach acid

____ 25.   Increase lower esophageal sphincter tone and help empty the stomach

____ 26.   Treat *H. pylori* infections

A.   Cytoprotective drugs

B.   Proton pump inhibitors

C.   Histamine H_2 blockers

D.   Antibiotics

E.   Antacids

F.   Promotility drugs

MEDICATION SAFETY PRACTICE

1. Patients taking large doses of antacids containing calcium or aluminum salts over a long period of time are at risk for developing _____.

2. Patients taking Milk of Magnesia for indigestion over a long period of time are likely to develop _____.

3. Antacids such as Alka-Seltzer or Bromo-Seltzer are contraindicated for patients who have _____ _____.

4. Bismuth subsalicylate (Pepto-Bismol) is contraindicated in children because of the risk for developing _____ _____.

5. A patient is to take 15 mL of Maalox at bedtime. What is the household equivalent of this dose? _____

PRACTICE QUIZ

1. Which lab tests are monitored for patients who are taking nizatidine (Axid) or cimetidine (Tagamet)? *(Select all that apply.)*
    ____ A. Complete blood count
    ____ B. Liver function tests
    ____ C. Electrolytes
    ____ D. Urinalysis
    ____ E. Pulmonary function tests

____ 2. A 14-year-old patient who weighs 143 pounds is prescribed clarithromycin (Biaxin) for *H. pylori* infection. The recommended children's dose is 15 mg/kg orally in 2 divided doses. What is the correct dose in milligrams for *each* of the doses given in one day? _____ mg

3. Long-term use of proton pump inhibitors can lead to which conditions? *(Select all that apply.)*
    ____ A. Gastric infections
    ____ B. Bowel obstruction
    ____ C. Drowsiness
    ____ D. Anemia
    ____ E. Halitosis

____ 4. Which statement demonstrates a patient's understanding of therapy with cytoprotective drugs for treatment of GERD?
    A. "I will take this medicine until it relieves my symptoms."
    B. "This drug will be a lifelong treatment for my stomach problems."
    C. "I need to keep my vegetable and fruit intake down while I'm on this medication."
    D. "I must take this drug for as long as my doctor prescribes it."

____ 5. During a follow-up assessment of a patient taking metoclopramide (Reglan) for treatment of GERD, you observe an elevated temperature, respiratory distress, tachycardia, diaphoresis, and urinary incontinence. What is the priority action for this situation?
    A. Check the patient's medical record for drug allergies.
    B. Notify the prescriber.
    C. Give the antidote for metoclopramide.
    D. Place the patient on a cooling blanket.

____ 6. An older adult has been prescribed cimetidine (Tagamet). What is a lifespan consideration for this patient?
   A. A black tongue or bowel movement is a common effect of this medication.
   B. Due to decreased calcium absorption, hip fractures are more common.
   C. Older adults are more likely to experience dizziness and confusion.
   D. This patient should be taught how to avoid excessive exposure to the sun.

____ 7. A patient asks how the proton pump inhibitor lansoprazole (Prevacid) will help the symptoms of GERD. How does the nurse respond?
   A. "It prevents stimulation of the pumps in your stomach that produce acid."
   B. "It blocks the action of acid-secreting cells in your stomach."
   C. "It neutralizes acids in your stomach to decrease irritation."
   D. "It coats the mucosal lining of your stomach."

____ 8. Which patient statement best indicates a correct understanding of why the antibiotic clarithromycin (Biaxin) has been prescribed along with another medication for ulcers?
   A. "It treats infection with *H. pylori*."
   B. "It is effective against inflammation in the stomach."
   C. "It prevents peritonitis in the event of stomach perforation."
   D. "It treats fever associated with neuroleptic malignant syndrome."

____ 9. A patient has been taking metoclopramide (Reglan) for several months to treat GERD. The patient is noted to have uncontrolled jerking–type movements of the mouth and face. She is puckering her lips, and has rapid movements of the tongue. These symptoms are consistent with the development of which adverse effect of the medication?
   A. Perforation of a peptic ulcer
   B. Neuroleptic malignant syndrome
   C. Tardive dyskinesia
   D. Parkinson's disease

____ 10. An older adult will be taking metoclopramide (Reglan) to treat symptoms of GERD. Which safety instruction is most crucial to provide?
   A. "You must stop driving altogether."
   B. "Never eat spicy or greasy foods again."
   C. "This drug may increase your blood pressure."
   D. "Sit up slowly from a resting position."

____ 11. You are assisting a patient to set up a schedule for taking sucralfate (Carafate) to treat an ulcer. Which is the most appropriate schedule for this medication?
   A. Every 6 hours around the clock
   B. One hour before meals and at bedtime
   C. An hour after meals and at bedtime
   D. With each meal and then at bedtime

____ 12. A patient is taking bismuth subsalicylate (Pepto-Bismol) to treat an ulcer. The patient reports having constipation, gray-black stools, and a gray-colored tongue. What is the most likely explanation of this?
   A. These are common side effects of the medication.
   B. These indicate nonhealing of the ulcer.
   C. These are symptoms of gastrointestinal bleeding.
   D. The patient is exceeding the prescribed dose.

Drug Therapy with Nutritional Supplements

chapter

24

LEARNING ACTIVITIES

Matching

Match the mineral/vitamin with the possible effects of its deficiency.

_____ 1. Folic acid

_____ 2. Cyanocobalamin

_____ 3. Thiamine

_____ 4. Niacin

_____ 5. Ascorbic acid

_____ 6. Vitamin D

_____ 7. Vitamin K

_____ 8. Calcium

A. Beriberi
B. Pellagra
C. Scurvy
D. Spina bifida in the fetus
E. Rickets
F. Osteoporosis
G. Bleeding, bruising
H. Megaloblastic anemia

Fill in the Blank

9. A deficiency of fluoride can lead to _____ _____, _____ _____, and _____.

10. _____, _____, _____, and _____ _____ are foods that contain iodine.

11. A patient with iron deficiency anemia could supplement the diet with which foods? (List four.)

_____

_____

_____

_____

12. To improve wound healing, a patient is advised to increase dietary zinc intake by including which foods in the diet? (List four.)

_____

_____

_____

_____

13. A patient who has an iodine deficiency is prone to developing

_____.

14. A diet can be sufficient in vitamin K with the intake of which foods? (List two.)

_____

_____

15. To prevent ascorbic acid deficiency, a patient can consume these foods: _____, _____, and

_____.

MEDICATION SAFETY PRACTICE

1. In the clinic, you observe a parent tell a child, "Now it's time for you to eat your candy," when referring to a chewable multivitamin. What is the concern with this action?

2. What are the signs associated with a severe allergic reaction to a vitamin/mineral supplement?

3. A patient is taking a mineral supplement containing potassium. What food seasoning should the patient avoid?

4. A patient who is receiving enteral nutritional supplement has diarrhea. What complication can result?

5. To prevent organism growth and infection, it is recommended to change enteral feeding containers and tubing how frequently?

PRACTICE QUIZ

_____ 1. The nurse is working with a new employee while caring for a patient receiving enteral nutritional supplements. The employee should be corrected if he attempts which action?
A. Hanging only 4 hours volume of supplement at a time.
B. Placing the head of the bed flat while the supplement is running.
C. Flushing the tube after feedings to prevent clogging of the tube.
D. Monitoring the patient's weight on a daily basis, using the same scale.

_____ 2. The health care provider has just inserted a nasogastric tube at the patient's bedside. What should be the nurse's next action?
A. Wait until an X-ray can confirm correct placement.
B. Begin infusing clear liquids through the tube.
C. Prepare for insertion of a central venous access device.
D. Place the head of the bed at a 15-degree angle.

_____ 3. Which is a common reason a patient is receiving total parenteral nutrition?
A. The patient has prolonged anorexia.
B. The patient has sustained a burn injury.
C. The patient has lost small intestine function.
D. The patient is experiencing a coma.

_____ 4. Which symptom is associated with potassium deficiency?
A. Goiter, swelling in the neck
B. Joint pain and stiffness
C. Anemia, shortness of breath
D. Muscle cramping and weakness

_____ 5. A patient who has been taking iron supplements for about a week reports black stools. What should be the nurse's action?
A. Recognize this is a sign of gastrointestinal bleeding.
B. Remind the patient this is expected and not harmful.
C. Assess the patient further for signs of an allergic reaction.
D. Advise the patient to consider discontinuing the medication.

_____ 6. An older adult woman wants to know why her health care provider recommended calcium supplements. What is the best explanation?
A. Calcium prevents megaloblastic anemia.
B. Calcium prevents bone cancer.
C. Calcium prevents osteomyelitis.
D. Calcium prevents osteoporosis.

_____ 7. A patient has been advised to increase calcium intake. Which item selected by the patient best demonstrates understanding of the instructions?
A. Canned salmon with bones
B. Baked tilapia with lemon
C. Shrimp tacos with lime juice
D. Fried catfish and coleslaw

_____ 8. Due to religious and cultural beliefs, a patient follows a strict vegan diet. Which foods will help improve the patient's iron intake?
A. Oranges, bananas, and grapefruit
B. Dried legumes and mustard greens
C. Milk, cheese, and yogurt
D. Chocolate and hard drinking water

_____ 9. Which is a common reason an older adult has a multivitamin supplement prescribed?
A. To assist in the absorption of prescribed medications
B. To prevent toxicities caused by prescribed medications
C. A decreased appetite can prevent getting enough essential vitamins
D. To decrease overall use of antacids when treating gastroesophageal reflux disease

10. Which vitamins are considered water-soluble? *(Select all that apply.)*

____ A.   Vitamin A

____ B.   Vitamin D

____ C.   Vitamin B_{12}

____ D.   Vitamin C

____ E.   Vitamin K

____ 11. Through which device can total parenteral nutrition be administered?

A.   Central venous access

B.   Nasogastric tube

C.   Nasojejunal tube

D.   Gastrostomy tube

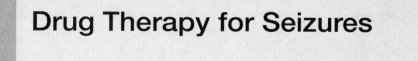

Drug Therapy for Seizures

chapter

25

LEARNING ACTIVITIES

Crossword Puzzle: Common Drug Names

Complete the puzzle by identifying the trade names of the antiseizure drugs that are described below in generic form.

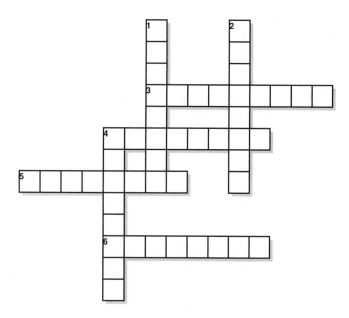

Across

3. gabapentin
4. valproic acid
5. primadone
6. carbamazepine

Down

1. clonazepam
2. ethosuximide
4. phenytoin

Matching: Terminology Review

Match the descriptions on the right with their correct terms on the left. (Answers will be used only once.)

____ 1.	Epilepsy	A.	Blank stare, chewing movements, lasting less than 29 seconds
____ 2.	Myoclonic seizure	B.	Sudden loss of muscle tone followed by confusion
____ 3.	Seizure	C.	Tingling, smell, or emotional changes occurring before a seizure
____ 4.	Partial seizure	D.	Brain disorder causing recurrent unprovoked seizures
____ 5.	Aura	E.	Electrical discharges from both sides of the brain
____ 6.	Status epilepticus	F.	Brief muscle jerk due to abnormal brain activity
____ 7.	Absence seizure	G.	Abnormal brain activity that starts in one part, may spread to the entire brain
____ 8.	Tonic-clonic seizure	H.	Interval following a seizure featuring confusion, headache, and fatigue
____ 9.	Atonic seizure	I.	Uncontrolled brain activity that may result in physical convulsion
____ 10.	Postictal phase	J.	Prolonged seizure or series of repeated seizures in a short interval
____ 11.	Generalized seizure	K.	Stiffening or rigidity of arm and leg muscles with loss of consciousness

Fill in the Blank

List the medical term for each side effect of antiseizure medication below.

12. Loss of coordination, clumsiness:_____

13. Double vision: _____

14. Involuntary movements of the eyes: _____

15. Excessive growth of gum tissue:_____

16. Low platelet count: _____

17. Low white blood cell count: _____

Matching: Second-Line (Alternative) Drugs for Seizures

Match the descriptions on the right with the correct drugs on the left. (Answers will be used only once.)

____ 18.	clonazepam (Klonopin)	A.	Blocks or slows the spread of abnormal electrical impulses
____ 19.	gabapentin (Neurontin)	B.	Turns into phenobarbital in the body and blocks or slows the spread of abnormal electrical impulses
____ 20.	phenobarbital (Luminal)	C.	Stabilizes the membranes of neurons to decrease seizure activity
____ 21.	primidone (Mysoline)	D.	Action not well understood but most likely slows or stops transmission of abnormal electrical impulses

MEDICATION SAFETY PRACTICE

_____ 1.   What can the nurse do to reduce nausea and vomiting in a patient who
        is taking carbamazepine (Tegretol)?
        A.   Give the medication early in the morning, before breakfast.
        B.   Administer the drug at bedtime.
        C.   Give the medication with food.
        D.   Give the drug with an antacid.

2.   Which are essential aspects of care for a patient who is experiencing a
        tonic-clonic seizure? _(Select all that apply.)_
        _____ A.   Help the person to the floor.
        _____ B.   Loosen clothing around the neck.
        _____ C.   Place a padded tongue blade in the mouth.
        _____ D.   Turn the person to the side.
        _____ E.   Remove any sharp objects.
        _____ F.   Administer an immediate oral dose of antiseizure medication.

_____ 3.   Which two drugs that are given to control seizures may become habit-
        forming?
        A.   Carbamazepine (Tegretol) and valproic acid (Depakote)
        B.   Phenytoin (Dilantin) and ethosuximide (Zarontin)
        C.   Primidone (Mysoline) and lamotrigine (Lamictal)
        D.   Phenobarbital (Luminal) and clonazepam (Klonopin)

4.   An older adult is more likely to experience which adverse effect from a
        first dose of phenytoin?

5.   Although many drugs to treat seizures are considered category C or D,
        what are the risks to mother and fetus if a seizure occurs during preg-
        nancy?

PRACTICE QUIZ

_____ 1.   Which statement demonstrates a patient's
        understanding of therapy with valproic
        acid (Depakote)?
        A.   "As soon as I stop having seizures, I
             will quit taking these pills."
        B.   "If I miss a dose, I need to take it as
             soon as possible, but not if it would
             be doubling a regularly scheduled
             dose."
        C.   "Since I have partial seizures, I only
             need to take part of one of these tab-
             lets."
        D.   "If I notice slowed wound healing, I
             will call my doctor right away."

_____ 2.   A patient taking phenytoin should be in-
        structed to call the prescriber immediate-
        ly if he or she develops what condition?
        A.   Excessive growth of hair in areas not
             normally hairy
        B.   Overgrowth of gum tissue
        C.   Difficulty coordinating movements
        D.   Drowsiness

____ 3. The health care facility should plan to have which drug immediately available in the event a patient experiences status epilepticus?
A. Diazepam (Valium)
B. Phenytoin (Dilantin)
C. Carbamazepine (Tegretol)
D. Valproic acid (Depakote)

____ 4. Good oral hygiene is important for patients who are taking phenytoin (Dilantin) over long periods of time because of what side effect?
A. Diplopia
B. Nystagmus
C. Hypertrichosis
D. Gingival hyperplasia

____ 5. Which consideration is most important to remember for adolescents who are taking a first-line drug for generalized seizures?
A. They often require decreased doses because of growth changes.
B. They often require decreased doses because of hormonal changes.
C. Sometimes they stop taking the medication to avoid gum changes.
D. They often take extra doses to avoid noticeable skin changes.

____ 6. Which instruction is most appropriate for the nurse to teach a pregnant patient who is taking a second-line drug for seizures?
A. Dizziness is more common when taking lamotrigine (Lamictal).
B. Reduce your folic acid intake when taking lamotrigine (Lamictal).
C. Primidone (Mysoline) may cause clotting problems in newborns.
D. Phenobarbital (Luminal) is associated with large-for-gestational-age fetuses.

____ 7. The nurse is obtaining a list of home medications for a patient who will be taking phenytoin (Dilantin) and an anticoagulant. What is the possible interaction between these two drugs?
A. The effect of anticoagulants is decreased.
B. Phenytoin tends to block the effect of anticoagulants.
C. The dosage of phenytoin may need to be increased.
D. The patient is at higher risk for bleeding.

____ 8. A patient experiences a seizure that lasts longer than 30 minutes. This situation is recognized as what kind of seizure?
A. Complex seizure
B. Status epilepticus
C. Partial seizure with secondary generalization
D. Myoclonic seizure

____ 9. A patient taking an antiseizure drug should avoid which food item?
A. Salted, cured bacon
B. Grapefruit juice
C. Eggs fried in butter
D. High-fiber oatmeal

____ 10. A patient taking valproic acid (Depakote) has developed a nosebleed and bruises resulting from very minor injuries. This patient may be developing which adverse effect?
A. Reduced red blood cells
B. Increased white blood cells
C. Increased red blood cells
D. Reduced platelet count

____ 11. During the transfer process between facilities, a patient's prescription for phenytoin (Dilantin) was overlooked. What consequence could occur to the patient?
A. The patient could develop seizures.
B. The patient's postictal stage is prolonged.
C. A more intense aura could occur.
D. Drug withdrawal symptoms are noted.

12. Which are possible consequences of exposure to phenytoin (Dilantin) during pregnancy? *(Select all that apply.)*
    ____ A. Drug withdrawal syndrome
    ____ B. Longer-than-normal fingernails
    ____ C. Increased risk for cleft palate
    ____ D. Growth deficiencies
    ____ E. Skull abnormalities

____ 13. A patient who takes carbamazepine (Tegretol) is discussing an upcoming vacation to a sunny beach location. Which special instruction is most crucial to provide for this patient?
    A. Drink plenty of water to avoid dehydration.
    B. Avoid overexertion with beachside sports.
    C. Wear sunscreen to avoid skin sensitivity.
    D. Increase the dosage to prevent stress-related seizures.

____ 14. A patient will be taking an antacid to deal with heartburn symptoms. She is also taking phenytoin (Dilantin) to treat seizures. How can the nurse best help the patient schedule use of these medications?
    A. Give the phenytoin 3 hours before taking the antacid.
    B. To simplify the schedule, give the medications at the same time.
    C. Give the antacid, then give the phenytoin 1 hour later.
    D. Suggest to the patient that she decrease the antacid dose by half.

Drug Therapy for Alzheimer's and Parkinson's Diseases

LEARNING ACTIVITIES

Matching

Match each generic drug name on the right with its correct trade name on the left. (Answers will be used only once.)

____ 1. Namenda

____ 2. Aricept

____ 3. Exelon

____ 4. Reminyl

A. galantamine
B. rivastigmine
C. memantine
D. donepezil

Matching: Drug Categories

Match each category of drug on the right with the correct drug on the left. (Categories will be used more than once.)

____ 5. entacapone (Comtan)

____ 6. selegiline (Eldepryl)

____ 7. pramipexole (Mirapex)

____ 8. apomorphine (Apokyn)

____ 9. tolcapone (Tasmar)

____ 10. rasagiline (Azilect)

____ 11. benztropine (Cogentin)

____ 12. ropinirole (Requip)

____ 13. trihexyphenidyl (Artane)

____ 14. bromocriptine (Parlodel)

____ 15. carbidopa/levodopa (Sinemet)

A. Dopamine antagonist
B. COMT inhibitor
C. MAO-B inhibitor
D. Anticholinergic

Matching: Key Terms

Match the key term with its definition. (Answers will be used once.)

_____ 16. A progressive, incurable condition that destroys brain cells, gradually causing loss of intellectual abilities

_____ 17. The loss of intellectual functions of sufficient severity to interfere with a person's daily functioning

_____ 18. A unique type of cell found in the brain and body that is specialized to process and transmit information

_____ 19. A chemical substance that transmits nerve impulses across a synapse

_____ 20. A progressive disorder of the nervous system marked by muscle tremors, muscle rigidity, decreased mobility, stooped posture, slowed voluntary movements, and a masklike facial expression

A. Neuron
B. Alzheimer's disease
C. Dementia
D. Neurotransmitter
E. Parkinson's disease

Fill in the Blank

21. Cholinesterase/acetylcholinesterase inhibitors _____ the activity of the _____ acetylcholinesterase.

22. _____ _____ block cholinergic nerve impulses to help control muscle movements.

23. Dopaminergic/dopamine agonists increase the amount of _____ _____ in the brain.

24. Alzheimer's disease affects _____% of people over age 65, and as many as _____% of people over age 85.

25. Parkinson's disease most commonly begins between the ages of _____ and _____.

26. In Parkinson's disease, nerve cells degenerate in a part of the basal ganglia called the _____ _____.

MEDICATION SAFETY PRACTICE

_____ 1. Before administering apomorphine (Apokyn), the nurse should obtain appropriate equipment to administer the medication by which route?
A. Oral
B. Intravenous
C. Intramuscular
D. Subcutaneous

____ 2. Due to the progressive effects of Alzheimer's disease, what must the nurse assess in a patient with the disease before administering oral medication?
   A. Intake and output for the day
   B. Vital signs
   C. Ability to swallow
   D. Daily weight

____ 3. What must family and patients be taught about administration of timed-release forms of medication?
   A. Always give with food.
   B. Do not give with grapefruit juice.
   C. Do not open or crush.
   D. Take with at least one full glass of water.

4. A patient with Parkinson's disease is prescribed ropinirole (Requip) 0.5 mg PO. The drug is available in scored tablets of 0.25 mg. How many tablets are given to the patient? _____ tablet(s)

5. A family member asks the nurse for assistance with "sorting out and organizing" medications for a patient who has Alzheimer's disease. Which medication is being given for which disorder? AcipHex? Aricept?

PRACTICE QUIZ

____ 1. Which drug for Alzheimer's disease reduces the activity of the enzyme acetylcholinesterase that breaks down acetylcholine in the synapses of neurons?
   A. Memantine (Namenda)
   B. Galantamine (Reminyl)
   C. Entacapone (Comtan)
   D. Selegiline (Eldepryl)

2. A patient who is taking donepezil (Aricept) for Alzheimer's disease should be monitored for symptoms of which adverse effects? *(Select all that apply.)*
   ____ A. Seizures
   ____ B. Tachycardia
   ____ C. Atrial fibrillation
   ____ D. Muscle weakness
   ____ E. Weight gain

____ 3. A nursing assistant in a long-term care facility reports that a patient with Alzheimer's disease choked several times during breakfast this morning. Which action is best to take before giving sustained-release galantamine (Razadyne) to this patient?
   A. Crush the medication and place it in applesauce or softened ice cream.
   B. Determine which food the patient enjoys and open the capsule onto it.
   C. Assess the patient's swallowing ability before giving the medication.
   D. Obtain the patient's height and weight to determine caloric needs.

_____ 4. Which statement by a family member indicates a correct understanding about the use of memantine (Namenda) for Alzheimer's disease?
   A. "I will administer this medication on an empty stomach."
   B. "This medication is also available in a skin patch."
   C. "This should improve the ability to perform complex tasks."
   D. "I will keep the medication stored in a safe location."

_____ 5. An older woman with Alzheimer's disease is very frail, weighing only 94 pounds. The nurse is reviewing the patient's medication record and notes that donepezil (Aricept) 10 mg PO at bedtime has been prescribed. What is the best action to take?
   A. Administer the medication with food to avoid GI upset.
   B. Change the administration time to every morning.
   C. Ask the patient which food she would like the medication with.
   D. Consult with the prescriber about the drug dosage.

   6. A patient is ordered pramipexole (Mirapex) to be given in three divided doses for a daily total of 4.5 mg. How many mg will each individual dose be?
   _____ mg

_____ 7. A patient who is taking entacapone (Comtan) reports feeling weak and achy recently. What question should the nurse ask the patient next?
   A. "What color is your urine?"
   B. "Have you lost more than 5 pounds in the last month?"
   C. "Do you have a fever?"
   D. "What color are the whites of your eyes?"
   E. "Have you had a bowel movement today?"

_____ 8. A patient who is taking ropinirole (Requip) to treat Parkinson's disease should be watched carefully for which potentially dangerous effect?
   A. Episodes of falling asleep suddenly
   B. Malignant melanoma
   C. Dyskinesia
   D. Rhinorrhea

_____ 9. A patient who is taking selegiline (Eldepryl) proudly announces he will be attending a college graduation party for his grandson. Which item must the patient avoid while taking this medication?
   A. Beer
   B. White wine
   C. Potato chips
   D. Pretzels

_____ 10. An older adult who is taking medication for Parkinson's disease should be cautioned to use extra care when walking because of which drug response?
   A. An increased risk for bradykinesia
   B. Rapid increase in blood pressure
   C. Confusion and hallucinations
   D. Rhinorrhea and excessive drooling

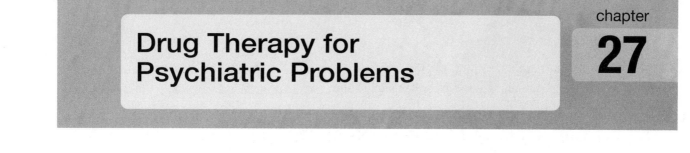

Drug Therapy for Psychiatric Problems

chapter **27**

LEARNING ACTIVITIES

Crossword Puzzle: Common Drug Names

Complete the crossword puzzle by identifying the correct trade names for each drug described below in generic form.

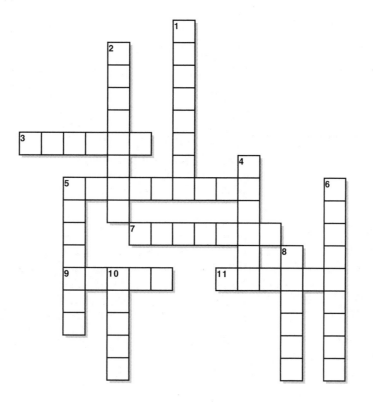

Across

3. fluoxetine
5. lithium carbonate
7. trazodone
9. paroxetine
11. thiothixene

Down

1. clonazepam
2. duloxetine
4. citalopram
5. escitalopram
6. risperidone
8. diazepam
10. alprazolam

Fill in the Blank

1. A selective serotonin reuptake inhibitor blocks the reuptake of
   _____, making it more available to act on _____
   in the brain.

2. Tricyclic antidepressants act by blocking the reuptake of _____
   and _____, making more of these substances available to act
   on receptors in the brain.

3. Other terms for an antipsychotic drug are _____
   _____ and _____.

4. Another term for an antianxiety drug is _____.

5. Neuroleptic malignant syndrome is associated with _____
   temperature, _____ pulse, _____,
   _____ respiratory rate, and _____ or
   _____ blood pressure.

Terminology Review

Match the descriptions on the right with their correct terms on the left. (Answers will be used only once.)

_____ 6. Anxiety

_____ 7. Bipolar disorder

_____ 8. Depression

_____ 9. Delusions

_____ 10. Dysthymia

_____ 11. Hallucinations

_____ 12. Illusions

_____ 13. Major depression

_____ 14. Mania

_____ 15. Obsessive-compulsive disorder

_____ 16. Panic disorder

_____ 17. Posttraumatic stress disorder

A. Alternating episodes of mania and depression
B. Fixed false beliefs or opinions that are resistant to reason
C. Feeling of dread about a perceived danger or threat
D. Incorrect mental representations of misinterpreted events
E. Feelings of sadness, despair, loss of energy, and difficulty coping
F. Sensory perceptions not actually present
G. Obsessive thoughts and compulsive actions
H. Persistently low moods; less severe than depression
I. Unexpected attacks of anxiety or terror lasting 15-30 minutes
J. Extremely elevated mood with mental and physical hyperactivity
K. Anxiety disorder caused by serious traumatic events
L. Persistent low mood and lack of pleasure in life with an increased risk of suicide

MEDICATION SAFETY PRACTICE

1. Patients taking venlafaxine, duloxetine, or bupropion are at risk for
   _____.

2. Patients on mirtazapine are at increased risk for infection because of
   _____.

3. Because of their abuse potential, _____ drugs are contraindicated for patients with a substance abuse disorder.

4. Patients taking quetiapine may experience an alteration in

_____ _____

_____.

5. A patient has been prescribed chlorpromazine (Thorazine) 35 mg IM STAT. The medication is available in vials of 50 mg/2 mL. How many mL should be administered to the patient? _____ mL

PRACTICE QUIZ

____ 1. A patient who has been taking the benzo-diazepine chlordiazepoxide (Librium) for anxiety reports after 2 weeks of therapy that she is feeling much calmer. This is a result of the enhanced inhibitory effects of which neurotransmitter?
A. Serotonin
B. Gamma-aminobutyric acid
C. Dopamine
D. Norepinephrine

____ 2. A patient who was prescribed lorazepam (Ativan) for 2 months suddenly stopped taking it because she "felt so much better." Now she reports restlessness, weakness, and insomnia. You should instruct her to call the prescriber and make an appointment immediately because of what risk associated with benzodiazepine withdrawal?
A. Sedation
B. Hypotension
C. Seizures
D. Stevens-Johnson syndrome

____ 3. A patient who is in her second trimester of pregnancy is experiencing emotional difficulty at home and asks her health care provider for a prescription for lorazepam (Ativan) to help her cope. Why is this drug contraindicated for this patient?
A. It can cause birth defects.
B. The fetus can become dependent on the drug.
C. The risk of preeclampsia is increased.
D. It might make the patient miscarry.

____ 4. A patient who has been taking sertraline (Zoloft) daily for 10 days reports that the medication has not helped with anxiety. What should the nurse tell the patient?
A. "This is a low dose and the prescriber will be contacted to request an increase."
B. "You should probably be taking a benzodiazepine for your condition."
C. "Another medication should be added to your regimen to get good results."
D. "You must give the drug more time because it is usually takes several weeks to be effective."

____ 5. A patient has begun treatment with 25 mg of chlorpromazine (Thorazine) BID. You should instruct the patient to be sure to practice which precaution?
A. Do not take the medication with grapefruit juice.
B. Record daily weights to monitor for retained fluid.
C. Change positions and get up slowly.
D. Check fasting blood sugar daily.

6. A patient has recently begun taking cita-lopram (Celexa) for symptoms of depression. You should monitor the patient for which common side effects? (Select all that apply.)
____ A. Insomnia
____ B. Anorexia
____ C. Dry mouth
____ D. Facial grimacing
____ E. Increased sweating

_____ 7. A group of individuals is participating in a support session to help with depression. Which patient statement would warrant an immediate notification of his or her health care provider?
   A. "I still have feelings of extreme sadness every single day."
   B. "When will this medication start to work? I still cry a lot."
   C. "My mouth is so dry, I wish I never started taking my medication."
   D. "If things don't improve, I'll have no reason to live anymore."

_____ 8. A patient who has taken chlorpromazine (Thorazine) has developed symptoms of muscle rigidity, elevated temperature, increased respiratory rate, and elevated pulse and blood pressure. In addition, the patient has become less responsive to verbal stimuli. Which adverse reaction has this patient developed?
   A. Tardive dyskinesia
   B. Neutropenia
   C. Neuroleptic malignant syndrome
   D. Myocarditis

_____ 9. Before giving clozapine (Clozaril) to a patient, you assess the patient's smoking history. What is the reason for this assessment?
   A. Hand tremors may cause self-injury while smoking.
   B. Smoking increases the risk of tardive dyskinesia.
   C. Smoking may decrease the effectiveness of clozapine.
   D. Smoking increases the risk of dementia.

_____ 10. Which statement made by a patient best indicates that the patient correctly understands the correct use of olanzapine (Zyprexa)?
   A. "I won't worry if this drug causes my urine to turn pinkish-brown."
   B. "I won't take this drug with grapefruit juice to avoid excessive blood levels."
   C. "I can drink a glass of wine at night to help me relax and sleep better."
   D. "Suntanning is acceptable, as long as I do not use a tanning bed."

_____ 11. An older adult has been taking lithium and develops nausea and vomiting. Which intervention is most appropriate?
   A. Contact the prescriber for possible parenteral fluids.
   B. Remind the patient to restrict fluid intake.
   C. Hold the lithium until the nausea subsides.
   D. Instruct the patient about ways to restrict sodium intake.

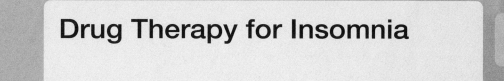

Drug Therapy for Insomnia

LEARNING ACTIVITIES

Crossword Puzzle

Complete the puzzle by identifying the correct terms that are described.

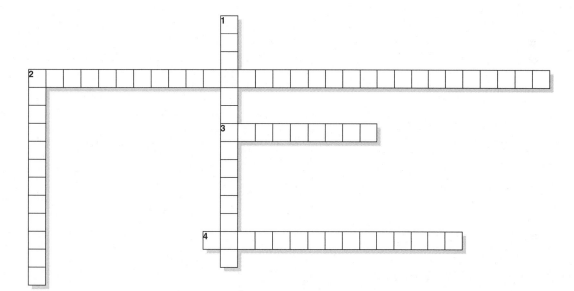

Across

2. A class of nonbenzodiazepine sedative-hypnotics that interacts with the same receptor site that benzodiazepine drugs do, turning on the receptors to induce sleep (three words)
3. Drugs that promote sleep by targeting signals in the brain to produce calm and ease agitation
4. A class of drugs that depress the CNS by binding to GABA receptors resulting in hypnotic and sedating effects; they are used mainly to control symptoms of anxiety or stress

Down

1. Drugs used to treat allergies and allergic reactions. Some, such as diphenhydramine (Allerdryl , Benadryl) and dimenhydrinate (Dramamine, Gravol), have sedating effects and are available over the counter
2. A class of drugs formed from barbituric acid that induces sedation and general depression over all CNS functions

Matching

Match each generic drug name on the right with its correct trade name on the left. (Answers will be used only once.)

_____ 1. Lunesta

_____ 2. Dalmane

_____ 3. ProSom

_____ 4. Restoril

_____ 5. Ambien

_____ 6. Sonata

_____ 7. Seconal

A. zolpidem
B. zaleplon
C. eszopiclone
D. flurazepam
E. estazolam
F. temazepam
G. secobarbital

Fill in the Blank

8. Benzodiazepines depress the CNS by binding to _____ _____.

9. _____ induce general depression over all CNS functions.

10. _____ and _____ function are inhibited by barbiturates.

11. Antihistamines produce _____ and _____ _____.

12. Drugs for insomnia are metabolized by the _____ and excreted by the _____.

MEDICATION SAFETY PRACTICE

1. A patient taking eszopiclone should be warned that serious adverse effects of this drug are _____ and _____ _____.

2. A patient with reduced liver function who is taking a drug to treat insomnia may have a(n) _____ drug level.

3. A patient has taken an overdose of a benzodiazepine. What is the reversal agent? _____ How is it administered? _____

4. A patient is to take 0.25 mg of triazolam (Halcion) at bedtime. The medication is available in 0.125-mg tablets. How many tablets should be administered? _____ tablets

5. Romazicon (Flumazenil) should not be given to a patient who has a(n) _____ _____.

PRACTICE QUIZ

____ 1. Benzodiazepines are prescribed for short-term treatment for which reason?
  A. They are excreted by the liver.
  B. They are formed from barbituric acid.
  C. They increase the seizure threshold.
  D. They are habit-forming.

____ 2. In addition to treatment for insomnia, barbiturates are used in management of which condition?
  A. Chronic pain
  B. Epilepsy
  C. Depression
  D. Psychosis

____ 3. Which intervention is most appropriate when administering a medication to treat insomnia?
  A. Remind the patient to change positions slowly.
  B. Administer the medication with a small glass of wine.
  C. Ask the patient to stay awake reading as long as possible.
  D. Leave extra medication at the bedside in case the patient wants another dose.

____ 4. A patient is taking a benzodiazepine receptor agonist for the first time at home. Which is the most appropriate instruction to give?
  A. Turn off all the lights in the house, and sleep alone.
  B. Take this medication about an hour before you go to bed.
  C. Have another person stay with you the first time you take this.
  D. Take this medication with an antihistamine, such as Benadryl.

____ 5. A patient requests information about taking zolpidem during an overnight airplane flight that lasts 5-6 hours. What information should the nurse provide?
  A. This may cause a transient memory loss.
  B. This is generally safe for most individuals.
  C. Wine or alcohol can improve the drug's effect.
  D. Stay awake during the flight, sleep upon arrival.

____ 6. A child will be taking chloral hydrate (Aquachloral) prior to a CT scan which requires the child to be very still. The child weighs 44 pounds. How many mg should the child receive? _____ mg

____ 7. A patient has had an overdose of a benzodiazepine. In addition to treatment with the reversal agent, the patient will need continued monitoring for which adverse effect?
  A. Increased excitability
  B. Respiratory depression
  C. Elevated blood pressure
  D. Myocardial infarction

____ 8. Which considerations apply to an older adult who is taking a drug to treat insomnia?
  A. A higher dose is usually necessary.
  B. Safety precautions are necessary to prevent falls.
  C. Drug addiction is more likely to occur.
  D. Older adults are less sensitive to side effects.

____ 9. A mother who is breastfeeding an infant requests information on drugs to treat insomnia. Which information is most appropriate to provide?
  A. These are usually safe to take while breastfeeding.
  B. The breastfed infant could be sedated by the medication.
  C. These drugs rarely enter into the breast milk.
  D. Take later at night to help you sleep better.

10. A patient will be taking flurazepam 30 mg this evening. The patient should be monitored for which common side effects? *(Select all that apply.)*
  ____ A. Excess energy
  ____ B. Restlessness
  ____ C. Daytime drowsiness
  ____ D. Blurred vision
  ____ E. Confusion

Drug Therapy for Eye Problems

LEARNING ACTIVITIES

Terminology Review

Match the descriptions on the right with the correct terms on the left. (Answers will be used only once.)

____ 1. Anterior chamber

____ 2. Anterior segment

____ 3. Aqueous humor

____ 4. Conjunctiva

____ 5. Glaucoma

____ 6. Miosis

____ 7. Mydriasis

____ 8. Posterior chamber

____ 9. Punctum

____ 10. Posterior segment

____ 11. Photoreceptors

____ 12. Retina

____ 13. Sclera

A. White outer layer of the eye
B. Clear membrane covering the front of the eye
C. Dilation of the pupil
D. Drains tears into the nasolacrimal sac
E. Back of the eye from the lens to the optic nerve
F. Increased intraocular pressure
G. Light-activated nerve endings
H. Clear fluid maintaining pressure and shape of the eye
I. Lining of the eye containing photoreceptors
J. Segment of the eye from the iris to the cornea
K. Constriction of the pupil
L. Part of the eye between the lens and the iris
M. Part of the eye between the lens and the cornea; contains chambers

Matching: Common Drug Names

Match the class of glaucoma drug on the right with the correct names on the left. (Types will be used more than once.)

____ 14. apraclonidine
____ 15. carbachol
____ 16. betaxolol
____ 17. bimatoprost
____ 18. acetazolamide
____ 19. levobunolol
____ 20. pilocarpine
____ 21. latanoprost
____ 22. methazolamide
____ 23. carteolol
____ 24. travoprost
____ 25. timolol
____ 26. dorzolamide
____ 27. echothiophate
____ 28. dipivefrin

A. Prostaglandin agonist
B. Beta blocker
C. Adrenergic agonist
D. Cholinergic
E. Carbonic anhydrase inhibitor

Matching: General Issues for Local Eye Drug Therapy

Indicate whether the following techniques or precautions should or should not be used for administration of drugs into the eye.

____ 29. Wash your hands before administering eye drugs.
____ 30. Remove contact lenses before applying eye drugs.
____ 31. Wash the eye with warm tap water before applying eye drugs.
____ 32. When two types of eyedrops are prescribed, mix them together and then apply.
____ 33. Before applying ointment, first squeeze out some of the ointment onto a tissue and discard it.
____ 34. Try to center the drop right over the pupil.
____ 35. After applying eyedrops, apply pressure over the patient's inner canthus.
____ 36. After applying eye ointment, tape the patient's eyelids closed for 1 hour.
____ 37. Teach patients to keep all eye ointments in the refrigerator (eyedrops can stay at room temperature).

A. Should use
B. Should not use

Matching: Drugs to Treat Glaucoma

Match the trade or brand name of each drug for glaucoma with its corresponding generic name. (Answers will be used once.)

____ 38. Diamox

____ 39. Iopidine

____ 40. Betoptic

____ 41. Lumigan

____ 42. Carboptic

____ 43. Propine

____ 44. Xalatan

____ 45. Betagan

____ 46. Ocusert

____ 47. Timoptic

____ 48. Travatan

A. timolol
B. latanoprost
C. betaxolol
D. apraclonidine
E. carbachol
F. dipivefrin
G. bimatoprost
H. levobunolol
I. pilocarpine
J. travoprost
K. acetazolamide

Fill in the Blank

49. An adrenergic agonist binds to the receptor sites in the eye that bind to naturally occurring _____ to reduce the amount of _____ humor produced.

50. _____ _____ _____ agents bind to adrenergic receptor sites and act as antagonists, preventing naturally occurring adrenalin from binding to the receptors.

51. _____ _____ _____ is a type of diuretic that lowers intraocular pressure by reducing production of aqueous humor.

52. A cholinergic agent increases the response that occurs when _____ binds to its receptor and activates it.

53. A prostaglandin agent binds to prostaglandin receptor sites in the eye, causing eye blood vessels to _____, allowing blood vessels to _____, draining more _____ _____.

MEDICATION SAFETY PRACTICE

____ 1. Why is aseptic technique used to instill eyedrops?
   A. The eye is sterile.
   B. Eye medications are sterile.
   C. The eye is not well-protected by the immune system.
   D. Drug interactions may occur when multiple medications are administered.

_____ 2. Some drugs for the eye are also available as regular topical ointments. How are these formulations different?
   A. Neither preparation is sterile.
   B. The drug concentration in topical ointments is lower.
   C. Topical ointments are suspended in non–water-soluble carriers.
   D. The particles contained in the topical ointments are larger and should not be put in the eye.

3. The action performed to reduce systemic absorption of eye medication is known as _____ _____.

4. Prostaglandin agonists should only be used if the eye is _____.

5. Long-term use of beta blockers can increase the risk for _____.

6. In patients who have asthma or heart failure, _____ _____ drugs should be used with caution.

7. Patients who have taken MAO inhibitors within the last 2 weeks should not use _____ _____ eye medications.

8. If a patient is to be administered another eye medication after a carbonic anhydrase inhibitor, there should be an interval of _____ between instilling the two drugs.

PRACTICE QUIZ

_____ 1. When an eye appears "bloodshot," the vessels that are visible are in what part of the eye?
   A. Sclera
   B. Pupil
   C. Aqueous humor
   D. Conjunctiva

_____ 2. An older adult patient with diabetes who is taking beta blockers for glaucoma must be instructed to perform what assessment?
   A. Daily weight
   B. Intake and output
   C. Blood glucose level
   D. Urine ketones

_____ 3. Which is most important to assess before administering a prostaglandin agent to a patient?
   A. Corneal color changes
   B. Excessive eyelash growth
   C. Presence of cataracts
   D. Whether the eye surface is intact

_____ 4. What teaching point must be included for a patient who is taking cholinergic drugs for treatment of glaucoma?
   A. Wear sunglasses when reading fine print indoors.
   B. Limit your fluid intake to less than 2000 mL per day.
   C. Apply punctal pressure for 10 minutes to avoid systemic effects.
   D. Use caution in dim lighting to prevent falls and injury.

_____ 5. A patient had an allergic reaction to a sulfa antibiotic 1 year ago. This indicates that the patient may have sensitivities to which eye medication?
   A. Carbonic anhydrase inhibitors
   B. Cholinergics
   C. Prostaglandin agonists
   D. Adrenergic blockers

____ 6. The rationale for pressing on the inner canthus after instilling eyedrops is to avoid what event?
   A. Overdosage
   B. Contamination
   C. Systemic side effects
   D. Increased intraocular pressure

____ 7. A middle-aged patient with glaucoma is not following the prescribed regimen for instilling eyedrops. He says he can see just fine and his eyes do not hurt. What factors regarding glaucoma should be reviewed with him?
   A. Vision damage from glaucoma occurs painlessly.
   B. When the pain from glaucoma returns, resume eyedrop use.
   C. When difficulty seeing occurs, resume eyedrop use.
   D. Your central vision would be affected first with glaucoma.

____ 8. A patient has been taught how to apply bimatoprost (Lumigan) eyedrops to treat glaucoma in the affected right eye. Which patient action indicates the need for further teaching?
   A. The patient administers the correct number of drops to both eyes.
   B. The drops are applied to the pocket of the lower lid of the eye.
   C. The patient avoids touching the eye with the tip of the bottle.
   D. The patient wipes away excess drops from the face with a tissue.

____ 9. Which assessment finding is most likely associated with use of travoprost (Travatan) for several months?
   A. Cloudiness of the lens
   B. Bulging of the eye tissues
   C. Darkening of the iris
   D. Unequal pupil size

____ 10. A patient has been taking timolol (Timoptic) eyedrops for several months and recently experienced a decreased pulse and worsening of asthma symptoms. What is the most likely explanation for this?
   A. The patient took the timolol orally, instead of adminstering to the eyes.
   B. The patient used the drops in both eyes instead of just one.
   C. The patient abruptly stopped using the prescribed eyedrops.
   D. The patient did not apply pressure to the punctum after administration.

Drug Therapy for Osteoporosis, Arthritis, and Skeletal Muscle Relaxation

chapter

30

LEARNING ACTIVITIES

Crossword Puzzle

Complete the puzzle by identifying the correct terms described in the clues below.

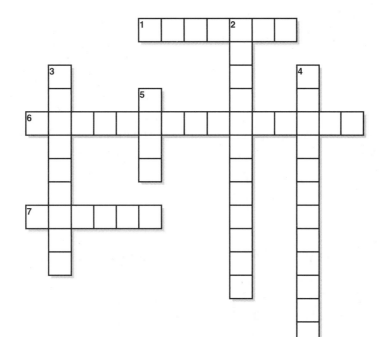

Across

1. Skeletal muscles require stimulation from the _____ system.
6. The generic names of the _____ have the syllable "dron" in the middle.
7. To straighten the bones around a joint, the _____ muscles relax.

Down

2. An increased risk for bone fractures is associated with _____.
3. Cyclobenzaprines are similar in structure to the _____ antidepressants.
4. _____ activity is replacement with new bone cells.
5. Excessive uric acid crystals can result in _____, a joint problem.

Matching

Match each drug on the left with its correct drug category on the right. (Some drug categories may be used more than once.)

____ 1. denosumab (Prolia)

____ 2. alendronate (Fosamax)

____ 3. ibandronate (Boniva)

____ 4. estrogen/bazedoxifene (Duavee)

____ 5. risedronate (Actonel)

____ 6. raloxifene (Evista)

____ 7. zoledronic acid (Reclast)

A. Bisphosphonates
B. Estrogen agonists/antagonists
C. Monoclonal antibodies

Matching

Match each drug on the left with its correct drug category on the right. (Some drug categories may be used more than once.)

____ 8. carisoprodol (Soma)

____ 9. allopurinol (Zyloprim)

____ 10. febuxostat (Uloric)

____ 11. rasburicase (Elitek)

____ 12. cyclobenzaprine (Flexeril)

A. Uric acid synthesis inhibitor
B. Enzyme, treats hyperuricemia, gout
C. Carbamates
D. Cyclobenzaprine

Fill in the Blank

13. _____ both prevents bones from losing calcium and increases bone density.

14. Carbamates act centrally to depress most CNS activity and reduce motor neuron depolarization, which leads to _____ _____.

15. Cyclobenzaprines change the influence of _____ in the spinal cord, which reduces _____ _____ _____, leading to skeletal muscle relaxation.

16. _____ _____ _____ is a drug category composed of antibodies directed against immature osteoclasts.

17. Uric acid synthesis inhibitors prevent the formation of uric acid, preventing _____.

MEDICATION SAFETY PRACTICE

1. A family member of an older couple approaches the nurse, asking for assistance in "sorting out" both parents' medications. There are bottles of Fosamax and Flomax. What is each medication prescribed for?

   Fosamax _____

   Flomax _____

2. In a similar situation, the bottles are Actonel and Actos. What is each medication prescribed for?

   Actonel _____

   Actos _____

3. Raloxifene (Evista) should not be given to patients who at risk for which problems? (List three.)

   _____

   _____

   _____

4. A patient is to be receiving an osteoclast monoclonal antibody today. Which adverse effect could occur with this drug? What precautions should be taken?

5. A patient who is African American should not receive which drug used to treat gout?

PRACTICE QUIZ

____ 1. The nurse is assisting with a patient's medication schedule. At which time should alendronate (Fosamax) be scheduled?
   A. Before breakfast
   B. With each meal
   C. After each meal
   D. At bedtime

____ 2. A patient will be receiving zoledronic acid (Reclast). Which administration technique is involved with administration of this medication?
   A. After administration, have the patient sit up for at least an hour.
   B. The medication is administered subcutaneously every month.
   C. The medication is administered intravenously once yearly.
   D. Before administration, ensure that bone marrow needles are available.

3. Which are the most common side effects of the bisphosphonates drug category? *(Select all that apply.)*
   ____ A. Muscle spasms
   ____ B. Abdominal pain
   ____ C. Skin rashes
   ____ D. Esophageal reflux
   ____ E. Nausea

____ 4. The nurse is assisting with scheduling medication administration for a patient who is to receive denosumab (Prolia). How should this medication be scheduled?
   A. Once every month
   B. Once every 3 months
   C. Once every 6 months
   D. Once every 12 months

____ 5. Which patient statement indicates the patient has understood instructions provided regarding allopurinol (Zyloprim)?
   A. "I'll need to take this on an empty stomach."
   B. "I'll need to drink plenty of water during the day."
   C. "This may turn my urine an orange-red color."
   D. "My gout is caused by overuse of my joints."

____ 6. A patient is receiving methocarbamol intravenously. What patient complaint should you report to the health care provider immediately?
   A. "I'm so sleepy I can hardly keep my eyes open."
   B. "I'm tired of waiting for that to infuse; speed it up."
   C. "My mouth is really dry; can you give me some water?"
   D. "My arm really hurts where the IV is going in."

____ 7. Cyclobenzaprine should not be given to a patient with which disorder?
   A. A fall resulting in back pain
   B. History of seizures
   C. Allergies to sulfa-type drugs
   D. Taking SSRIs to treat depression

____ 8. Carbamates are not recommended for older adults for which reason?
   A. There is an increased risk of myocardial infarction.
   B. The drug is considered less effective in older adults.
   C. The drug is more likely to be habit-forming in older adults.
   D. There is an increased risk for falls in older adults.

____ 9. Which is important to include in patient teaching for a patient taking a skeletal muscle relaxant?
   A. It is generally safe to take this medication with a small amount of alcohol.
   B. Do not drive or operate machinery while you are taking this medication.
   C. Sit down slowly from a standing position to prevent lightheadedness.
   D. This medication is generally taken for several months for muscle spasms.

____ 10. A patient is taking cyclobenzaprine (Flexeril) and mentions she has heard of "anticholinergic effects" from an article she read online. Which is an anticholinergic effect of this drug?
   A. Urinary frequency
   B. Visual hallucinations
   C. Having a dry mouth
   D. Diarrhea, loose stools

Drug Therapy for Male Reproductive Problems

chapter **31**

LEARNING ACTIVITIES

Crossword Puzzle: Terminology Review

Complete the puzzle by identifying the key terms that are described.

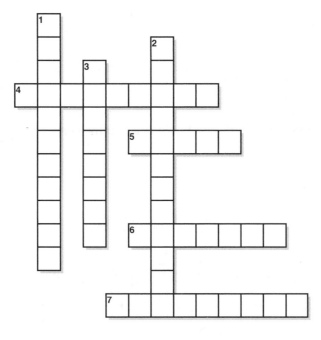

Across

4. The amount of circulating testosterone _____ with aging.
5. A reduced _____ of the urine stream is also a symptom of benign prostatic hyperplasia.
6. The prostate gland surrounds the upper part of the _____.
7. A symptom of benign prostatic hyperplasia is increased _____ of urination.

Down

1. Enlargement of the prostate gland is called benign prostatic _____.
2. Male hormone produced in the testes
3. A patient with benign prostatic hyperplasia should be seen by the health care provider to rule out _____ cancer.

Matching

Match each drug on the left with its correct drug category on the right. (Drug categories may be used more than once.)

_____ 1.   testosterone gel (AndroGel)

_____ 2.   dutasteride (Avodart)

_____ 3.   doxazosin (Cardura)

_____ 4.   tamsulosin (Flomax)

_____ 5.   testosterone patch (Androderm)

_____ 6.   terazosin (Hytrin)

_____ 7.   finasteride (Proscar)

_____ 8.   vardenafil (Levitra)

A.   DHT inhibitors
B.   Selective alpha$_1$ blockers
C.   Testosterone drugs
D.   Drugs for erectile dysfunction

Fill in the Blank

9.   List four symptoms of insufficient testosterone.

10. A patient who takes a DHT inhibitor should be advised that the herbal substances _____ _____ and
_____ _____ could have an increased intended drug response and increased side effects.

11. A patient taking a DHT inhibitor may experience a slowing of
_____ _____ from the scalp.

12. Selective alpha$_1$ blockers act to relax _____
_____ _____ in the prostate gland.

13. DHT inhibitors bind to the enzyme that normally converts
_____ to DHT.

14. The most common side effect of drugs for BPH is decreased
_____.

15. Tamsulosin may cause an allergic reaction in patients who are allergic to
_____ _____.

MEDICATION SAFETY PRACTICE

_____ 1. The nurse is working with a patient who is taking dutasteride (Avodart) 5 mg daily. The patient's granddaughter, who is in the second trimester of pregnancy, says she wants to cut the tablets in half so the patient can swallow them easily. What should be the nurse's response?
   A. "These can easily be broken in half. Just make sure to give him both halves."
   B. "You should not handle these tablets, especially when they are cut in half."
   C. "You need to move out of your grandfather's house while he is taking this drug."
   D. "If cutting them in half doesn't work, crush them and put them in applesauce."

2. A patient with impaired liver function should not take finasteride (Proscar) for which reason?

3. A patient is taking finasteride (Proscar) and states he is still sexually active with his wife, who is now pregnant. What special teaching is necessary?

4. A patient who is taking tamsulosin (Flomax) is having cataract eye surgery in a week. What problem can occur during this surgery?

5. Testosterone is pregnancy category _____.

PRACTICE QUIZ

_____ 1. A patient has been educated about taking his first dose of doxazosin (Cardura). What patient statement indicates the need for further instruction?
   A. "I'll take this medication at night, right before I go to bed."
   B. "I'll take this medication before I drive to work in the morning."
   C. "If I get dehydrated, I'm more likely to get dizzy when I stand up."
   D. "My son is staying with me the first night I take it, in case I need to get up."

_____ 2. An older male patient taking a drug for benign prostatic hyperplasia needs to visit his health care provider annually for which reason?
   A. Pharmacies will not renew the prescription without an annual refill order.
   B. Older adults are more likely to develop heart failure and hypertension.
   C. Prostate cancer is more likely to occur in males during the aging process.
   D. The drug tends to be less effective with aging and the dose needs to be increased.

____ 3. A patient is to receive an IM injection of testosterone cypionate 150 mg IM. The vial is labeled 200 mg/mL. What is the amount to be given? _____ mL

____ 4. Which assessment finding is a common side effect of treatment with testosterone?
A. Dry, scaly skin
B. Enlarged testicles
C. Pitting ankle edema
D. Breast enlargement

____ 5. Which patient should *not* receive treatment with testosterone?
A. A patient with a history of breast cancer
B. A patient with a decreased interest in sex
C. A patient with decreased bone density
D. A patient with depression and irritability

____ 6. To avoid virilization effects in women exposed to testosterone gel or patches, which precaution should be in place?
A. The clothing and linen used by the man should be hand-washed, not machine-laundered.
B. It is safe for the woman to apply the testosterone gel, as long as she washes her hands afterwards.
C. Avoid touching the skin, clothing, or linen that has been in contact with the testosterone gel.
D. The patch can be placed or removed by a female, as long as she washes her hands afterwards.

____ 7. Which is an organic risk factor for erectile dysfunction?
A. Depression
B. Diabetes
C. Anxiety
D. Stress

____ 8. Phosphodiestrase-5 inhibitor drugs help with erectile dysfunction in which manner?
A. Relax smooth muscles and allow the penis to fill with blood
B. Contract voluntary muscles to improve blood flow to the penis
C. Allow penile erection to occur in the absence of sexual stimulation
D. About 10 minutes after taking the drug, an erection is likely to occur

____ 9. A patient mentions having a headache after using sildenafil (Viagra). The patient can be advised to use the recommended dose of which medication to treat these symptoms?
A. Acetaminophen (Tylenol)
B. Hydrocodone (Norco)
C. Doxazosin (Cardura)
D. Sublingual nitroglycerine

10. A patient is taking a drug to treat BPH symptoms. Which indicate the medication is effective? *(Select all that apply.)*
____ A. Less difficulty starting the urine stream
____ B. A feeling of bladder fullness
____ C. A reduction in sexual libido
____ D. Needing to urinate less frequently at night
____ E. Improved overall body strength

____ 11. Which side effect of dutasteride (Avodart) has future reproductive implications?
A. Decreased fertility
B. Births of multiples
C. Increased libido
D. Increased seminal fluid

Drug Therapy for Female Reproductive Problems

LEARNING ACTIVITIES

Crossword Puzzle: Terminology Review

Complete the puzzle by identifying the key terms that are described.

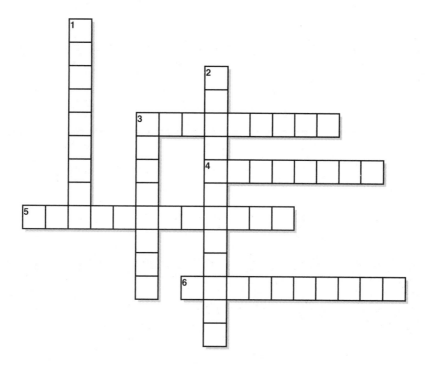

Across
3. The cessation of menstrual periods and ovulation
4. The main female sex hormone secreted by the ovaries
5. The periodic shedding of the uterine lining
6. The ovum is fertilized by a sperm

Down
1. The release of a mature ovum
2. The female hormone that supports pregnancy by maintaining the thickened uterine lining
3. The term for the beginning of the years of menstruation

Matching

Match the definition on the left with the correct term on the right. (Each answer will be used once.)

____ 1.   Shedding of the uterine lining

____ 2.   Beginning of the years of menstruation during adolescence

____ 3.   Interest in sexual activity

____ 4.   Cessation of menstrual periods and ovulation

____ 5.   Glandular cells in the ovary shrink and become nonfunctional

____ 6.   Transition between having regular menstrual cycles to time
          when menstrual periods have stopped for a full year

____ 7.   Blood vessels dilating, causing uncomfortable symptoms

____ 8.   Mature ovum is fertilized by a sperm

A. Menarche
B. Hot flashes
C. Menstruation
D. Perimenopause
E. Menopause
F. Libido
G. Pregnancy
H. Involution

Fill in the Blank

9. _____ is the main female hormone secreted by the ovaries
   and adrenal glands.

10. Follicle-stimulating hormone causes the ovary to secrete estrogen, allowing
    one ovum in the ovary to _____ _____
    each month.

11. _____ _____ causes secretion of proges-
    terone by the ovary and allows the release of a mature ovum.

12. Progesterone supports pregnancy by maintaining the thickened
    _____ _____.

13. Dropping levels of estrogen and progesterone allow the lining of the uterus
    to stop growing, and to be shed as _____.

14. If conception occurs, the fertilized ovum implants into the uterine lining
    within ____ to ____ days.

15. When the glandular cells of the ovary shrink, they no longer produce normal
    levels of _____.

MEDICATION SAFETY PRACTICE

1. Estrogen-based hormone replacement therapy is not recommended for long-
   term therapy due to which concern?

2. A patient who is considering use of estrogen-based hormone replacement
   therapy smokes. What advice should she be given, and why?

3. In women who still have a uterus and are taking perimenopausal HRT, the uterine lining can thicken, causing which problem?

4. Which type of cancers are hormone-sensitive and whose growth can be increased by perimenopausal HRT?

5. Perimenopausal HRT can increase the risk for which gastrointestinal disorders?

PRACTICE QUIZ

____ 1. A woman has been provided instructions on use of oral contraceptives. Which patient statement indicates the need for further instructions?
   A. "If I miss one dose, I should throw all the pills away, and start a new pack in a month."
   B. "I should plan on using a barrier method, such as a condom for the first month on the pill."
   C. "If I miss one dose within a cycle, the drug should still be effective to prevent pregnancy."
   D. "If I miss two doses, I should use another type of contraceptive while continuing the pill."

____ 2. A patient undergoing menopause asks, "How will I know if the hormone replacement therapy is working?" Which is the nurse's best response?
   A. "Your menstrual cycles will eventually become more regular."
   B. "Your symptoms of hot flashes and night sweats will lessen."
   C. "Your menstrual cycles will become less painful and less heavy."
   D. "Your symptoms of fluid retention and weight gain will improve."

____ 3. A patient has recently begun taking HRT. During subsequent visits, the patient should be assessed for which common side effect of HRT?
   A. Weight loss
   B. Facial hair growth
   C. Fluid retention
   D. Scalp hair loss

____ 4. A patient is to be monitored for liver dysfunction after beginning HRT. Which assessment findings are associated with liver dysfunction?
   A. Pale, waxy skin
   B. Oral cyanosis
   C. Yellow tinge to the skin
   D. Ruddy face

____ 5. A young adult requests information about various forms of contraception. Which form of contraception is most reliable?
   A. Oral contraceptive pills
   B. Implanted contraceptives
   C. Condoms and spermicides
   D. Complete abstinence

____ 6. Oral contraceptives are effective for which reason?
   A. The uterus lining sheds more often.
   B. Ovulation does not occur.
   C. Menstrual cycles are more frequent.
   D. The uterine lining thickens.

____ 7. A patient mentions she has heard of the "mini-pill" and requests information about this. What information should the nurse provide?
   A. It raises the blood level of progesterone.
   B. It decreases the blood level of estrogen.
   C. It is smaller and easier to swallow.
   D. It is to be taken only once a month.

____ 8. A patient is having her annual physical exam and renewal of her prescription of drospirenone (Yasmin). What is the most likely reason she is scheduled for a blood test today?
   A. To determine if she is using the medication as prescribed.
   B. To determine whether her potassium level is elevated.
   C. To determine if her estrogen levels are still sufficient.
   D. To determine if she has bone marrow cancer.

____ 9. A patient has been provided information about oral contraceptives. Which patient statement indicates the need for further education?
   A. "I'll need to take this medication at the same time every day."
   B. "I'll make sure to keep getting screened for cervical cancer."
   C. "I'm glad I won't be exposed to any sexually transmitted diseases."
   D. "I'll need to discuss any new medications with the provider."

____ 10. Children should not take either hormone replacement drugs or hormonal contraception before puberty for which reason?
   A. Its use has been associated with kidney disease.
   B. Children are more likely to develop breast cancer.
   C. Deep vein thrombosis is more likely to occur.
   D. This may cause growth of the long bones to stop.

____ 11. A mother who is breastfeeding her infant should not use hormonal contraception for which reason?
   A. It is likely to interfere with lactation.
   B. Breastfeeding is a natural contraceptive.
   C. It changes the contour of the breasts.
   D. It changes the breast milk flavor.